WEATHER
DISASTERS

WEATHER DISASTERS

HOW TO PREPARE FOR AND SURVIVE EARTHQUAKES, TORNADOES, BLIZZARDS, AND OTHER CATASTROPHES

MARK D. WILLIAMS AND AMY BECKER WILLIAMS

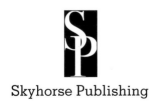

Skyhorse Publishing

Skyhorse Publishing books may be purchased in bulk at special discounts for sales promotion, corporate gifts, fund-raising, or educational purposes. Special editions can also be created to specifications. For details, contact the Special Sales Department, Skyhorse Publishing, 307 West 36th Street, 11th Floor, New York, NY 10018 or info@skyhorsepublishing.com.

Skyhorse® and Skyhorse Publishing® are registered trademarks of Skyhorse Publishing, Inc.®, a Delaware corporation.

Visit our website at www.skyhorsepublishing.com.

10 9 8 7 6 5 4 3 2 1

Library of Congress Cataloging-in-Publication Data is available on file.

Cover design by Tom Lau

Print ISBN: 978-1-5107-2862-2
Ebook ISBN: 978-1-5107-2863-9

Printed in China

TABLE OF CONTENTS

INTRODUCTION

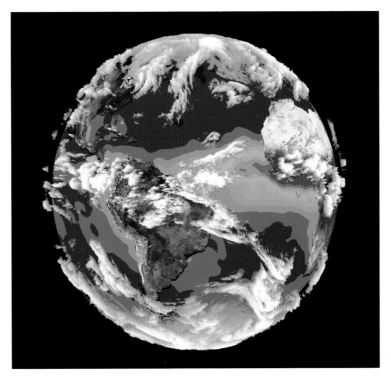

Satellite image of Earth's interrelated systems and climate. *Credit: NASA*

Severe weather events happen every day all over the world. We see the consequences on the evening news: tsunamis kill hundreds of thousands, mudslides ravage entire neighborhoods, floods devastate entire nations, and record hurricanes cause cataclysmic destruction throughout numerous islands. In 2017, America saw one of the most destructive hurricane seasons in its history. California endured one of its worst wildfire seasons ever.

We all are under threat from weather events no matter where we live, but rarely are we properly prepared. Like a New Year's Resolution, preparing for possible weather catastrophes sounds like a great idea, but the farther we move from it, the less likely it is we ever actually do it. We hope that this book sits on your table until that moment you decide to break the cycle and start preparing for the weather disaster most likely to affect you.

As we wrote these chapters, Houston was recovering from a thousand-year flood event at the hands of Hurricane Harvey, while Hurricane Irma had grown into a Category 5 and was bearing down on several Caribbean islands and ultimately, the American coast. Currently, weather events seem to be occurring with ever-increasing ferocity and strength. This holds true as Hurricane Irma is the strongest hurricane in the Atlantic basin outside of the Caribbean Sea and Gulf of Mexico in National Hurricane Center records. At the end of 2017, we even watched as a severe weather event we'd never heard of before unfolded off the Northeast Coast: the Bomb Cyclone.

These events are terrifying to witness and, in the wake of their power, people often feel helpless. This book, *Weather Disasters*, seeks to calm some of those fears and informs the reader how to prepare for, survive, and navigate through the aftermath of any major weather-related disaster. Given that earth is producing more and more frequent big weather events, many more once-in-a-century events, we hope this book is instructive and helpful with its timing. Think of all recent destructive disasters: Hurricane Katrina in 2005; the 2010 Haiti earthquake; the 2011 Japanese tsunami (at Fukushima Nuclear Plant); Superstorm Sandy 2012; and the record-setting 2017 seasons for Atlantic hurricanes and American wildfires. This book seems more relevant than ever. In addition to the above disasters, we include earthquakes and volcanoes since they affect weather and are similar in the amount of devastation that they can cause.

The weather disasters that typically cause the most deaths are hurricanes, earthquakes, and floods. All three are large events that can reach so much greater an area or region than can a tornado or landslide or avalanche. Tsunamis and volcano eruptions can also cause huge death tolls but, luckily, they don't happen often. Volcanoes may be the most destructive worldwide because they are climate-changers and species-killers but only erupt once every million years or so.

We should state upfront that we are not weather experts nor do we play ones on television. We simply are fans of weather and seasoned veterans of weather disasters, and so we wanted to put together a survival kit, so to speak, for bad weather. We have been through several kinds of bad weather and are nerdy enough to have put together loose plans and sorry disaster kits. But as severe storms became more common, we wanted to go deeper into survival planning and learn to do more for our family and property. In our own layman's fashion, we researched anything and everything.

We never planned to provide scientific detailed specifics on hurricanes or earthquakes and the like—there are books just for that, experts such as vulcanists, meteorologists, and seismologists who write deeply and intelligently about their subject. We set out to write an every-person's survival book for weather disasters. Our book is meant to introduce the best methods we found from our research on the best ways to prepare, to survive, and to manage the aftermath of the major weather and natural disasters. We're just normal folks who live in normal towns but still face risks from weather disasters. It'd be difficult to live anywhere in America without having to face one or more of these weather disasters—and in many places, several.

We have lived in Tornado Alley (Tornado Alley begins in central Texas and goes north through Oklahoma, central Kansas and Nebraska and eastern South Dakota, sometimes including the area east through Iowa, Missouri, Illinois, and Indiana to western Ohio) most of our respective fifty-seven and fifty-one years. We have been through dozens and dozens of tornado warnings, including at least five close calls where the storms came within a mile or less. We've lived in areas with extreme decade-long drought conditions. We have experienced hurricanes and blizzards. We've also experienced flash flooding, extreme lightning, wildfires, minor earthquakes, major hailstorms, and one particularly nasty haboob in Odessa, Texas in 1973. Mark visited Hawaii in the 1980s when the eruptions on the Big Island were especially common, devouring houses and destroying neighborhoods. At no point were we properly prepared or educated about any of the events we witnessed. We managed to avoid any human or property damage through no credit to us.

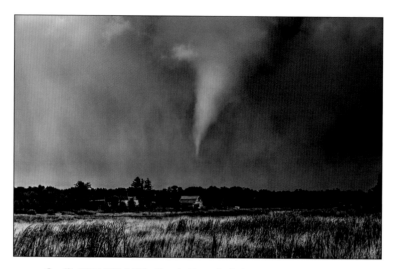

Credit: 2015 NOAA "Weather in Focus" photo contest, Amanda Hill.

Preparation is easy and is the most important part of weather-event survival. Survival is usually the result of preparation (with some luck) and a lot of remaining calm. The aftermath is often more deadly than the event—flooding, gas, contaminated water, unstable structures, etc. Warning fatigue is a dilemma we all face. We are inundated with so much information. Twenty-four-hour news channels, local news, newspapers, online news, smartphone notifications, and weather apps. Odds are that the hurricane will not hit you, the tornado will miss your house, and the earthquake won't happen this decade, but . . . this book is designed to help when it does. And weather disasters do happen to someone; one time soon it just might be you and your family. Education, preparation, and operation are the three key components of weather event survival. For each weather event you risk, you need the same conscientious action: make a plan and set up supplies. Decide how serious you are about your family's and property's safety. We are not trying to be cavalier about it. But we do want to be encouraging. A little prep goes a long way toward survival. Once you do it, you'll discover that it's comforting, useful, rewarding, sometimes fun, and most of all necessary, as it might save you and your family's lives.

ALERTS AND INFORMATION

It's a good time to remember: you won't be able to rely on your mobile device for everything. A handful of free emergency preparedness apps can help you in the event of a crisis even if you don't have cell service. Your local emergency response team will almost certainly offer several methods by which to get up-to-date information. They will generally tie into one or more radio stations, offer text messaging and social media sites, and be connected to both local television and the Red Cross.

Be careful about getting information from sources other than official sources and then re-tweeting or re-posting it. You might accidentally be forwarding information that is incorrect or only partly accurate, and that could be dangerous for others.

The Red Cross offers numerous apps, in fact, including the Shelter Finder app, First Aid, a hurricane app, an earthquake app, a wildfire app, and others. Each one includes checklists, advice for emergency situations (from performing first aid and CPR to handling food and water during power outages), quizzes, a sign-up for emergency notifications, and more. Facebook Check-In is also a useful emergency feature that, when activated because of a major disaster, allows users to inform friends and family of their whereabouts and safety status.

Similarly, the official FEMA (Federal Emergency Management Agency) website includes information for all kinds of disasters, including tips for creating an emergency kit, and emergency meeting locations, maps of important locations, and so on. Finally, the aptly-named Disaster Alert app offers a real-time map that shows active (or impending) incidents that have been deemed as "potentially hazardous to people, property, or assets." This includes hurricanes, floods, earthquakes, tsunamis, and volcanoes.

When planning for a disaster, there are certain persons that you need to keep in mind:

- **Children:** They rely on us for their well-being and safety. Keep them in mind when making plans. They are shorter, weaker, less educated and haven't seen many (if any) weather disasters. They will be scared, confused, and panicky. Water that's up to your knees might be neck-deep for them. Rushing water is scary to little ones. Earthquakes are nightmarish. Even for teenagers, weather disasters are frightening and disorienting. Our kids look to us for leadership. So if you include your children in your plans, allow them to have some ownership, educate them about the weather events and how these could play out, and generally show them that you are in charge, that there is a plan, and that everything will be okay. That's the role we have as adults and parents.

- **Disabled and elderly and needy:** People with access and functional needs require our planning and our assistance as much as children do. They might need adaptive equipment, means by which to power their electrical apparatus, help with transportation, medicines, and other needs.

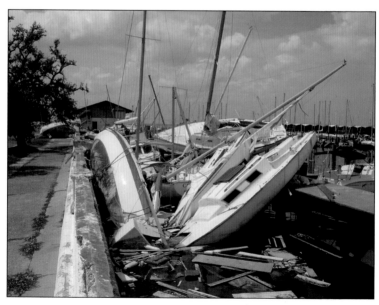

Hurricane damage after a 2005 storm. *Credit: Doug Helton, NOAA, NOS, ORR.*

Whether they are part of your family or neighborhood, be a part of their planning and survival.

- **Pets:** One of the saddest parts of our research was discovering how many pets are injured or killed because of weather-related events; the worst part is that most of the deaths could have been prevented by owners. Don't expect flooding and still leave your pet tied up outside. Don't expect blizzard conditions and leave your pet outside. Don't evacuate and not have made plans for your pet to survive. You took them in and they are part of your family. Treat them like it.

A universal checklist for your pet(s):

➢ Medications
➢ Important documents (vaccination records, medical history)
➢ Water and pet food (can opener if needed)
➢ Pet-friendly soap
➢ First-aid (triple antibiotic, Benadryl, etc.)
➢ Leash, collar, harness, muzzle
➢ ID tags
➢ Carrier if needed
➢ Current photo(s)
➢ Bowls for food and water
➢ Blanket or dog bed
➢ Litter and pan for cats
➢ Toys or treats

First Responders

If you think you might want to be a first responder, check with your local and community emergency organizations/agencies and see what roles are available and how to go about making it happen. A national emergency training program is called CERT (Community Emergency Response Team.) Check to see if your locale offers these courses, usually eight weeks in length. These awareness courses train people in basic disaster response skills such as fire suppression, urban search and rescue, and medical operations. CERT allows certified persons to take a more active role in emergency disaster response.

You might be instrumental in the planning aspect by setting up shelters and organizing neighborhoods. But if the disaster occurs and you're one of those with the determination to help others, be safe and don't take unnecessary chances. You can certainly be one of those heroes out in a boat fighting rising floodwaters and saving citizens and pets, but you can also be a hero by helping evacuate or attend to senior citizen homes, hospitals, and shelters. There are any number of ways to be a good citizen. Also, just to be neighborly, add to your inventory of supplies so you have them on hand when you go out to help others.

Layout of this Book

For each chapter, we break down the weather event into three parts: 1) Preparation; 2) Survival; and 3) Aftermath. We include conversational

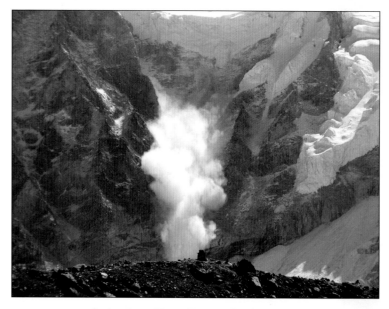

Avalanche on Mount Everest. *Credit: Pixabay.*

and informative narratives that feature the nature of this disaster, statistics of the event, sidebars and lists, and other relevant information. Each chapter also includes an emergency supply list and suggested items for a survival kit. There is a lot of crossover and repetition in each list, some basic emergency core necessities, but with each disaster, the list changes by addition. A volcano adds a respirator and goggles. Floods add wading boots. Some items you'll need for every list and they are indispensable. These are things we can't emphasize enough.

Ten Deadliest Natural Disasters

Rank is determined by estimated death toll

1. 1,000,000 to 4,000,000: 1931 China floods; China, July 1931
2. 900,000 to 2,000,000: 1887 Yellow River flood; China, September 1887
3. 830,000: 1556 Shaanxi earthquake; China, January 23, 1556
4. 300,000: 1839 India cyclone; India, November 26, 1839
5. 300,000: Calcutta Cyclone; India, October 7, 1737
6. 280,000: 2004 Indian Ocean earthquake and tsunami; Indian Ocean, December 26, 2004
7. 273,400: 1920 Haiyuan earthquake; China, December 16, 1920
8. 250,000 to 500,000; 1970 Bhola cyclone; East Pakistan (Bangladesh), November 13, 1970
9. 250,000 to 300,000: 526 Antioch earthquake; Byzantine Empire (Turkey), May 526
10. 242,000 to 655,000: 1976 Tangshan earthquake; China, July 28, 1976

CHAPTER ONE

HURRICANES

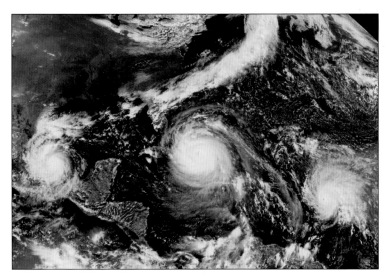

NOAA satellite of Hurricanes Katia, Irma, and José.

As we write this, we are witnessing the most astounding hurricane season in our history. There are three active hurricanes in the Atlantic at one time: Katia, Irma, and José. Irma is the strongest hurricane ever recorded in the Atlantic. Two weeks prior, Hurricane Harvey caused some $160 billion in damage, becoming the costliest hurricane on record, and caused the worst flooding hurricane in contiguous America's history with just under fifty-two inches of rain.

In an average year, North America and the Caribbean see twelve named tropical storms, six of which go on to become hurricanes. Three of those hurricanes will typically reach Category 3 or higher on the Saffir-Simpson Scale. In 2017, we saw seventeen named storms, ten of which strengthened into hurricanes and six of which reached Category 3 or stronger. While it was not a record-setting season in terms of the number of storms, it will likely be remembered as the one of the most intense, destructive, and costliest seasons in United States history. From Harvey's historic flooding of southeastern Texas, to the Irma-hammered Florida Keys and Maria's destruction in Puerto Rico, this series of major hurricanes wreaked havoc that will be felt for a decade.

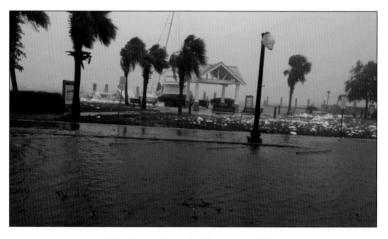

Hurricane Irma. *Credit: Eastern IMT.*

In one month's time, two Category 4 hurricanes, Harvey and Irma, made landfall, a rare occurrence. This was the first time two storms of such magnitude hit the American mainland in the same season since the early 1960s. Irma cut a swath through the Caribbean, smashing island after island on its course with Florida. Its width of four hundred-plus miles was bigger than the entirety of Florida itself. What most people will remember will be the second half of the season beginning with Franklin (August 6–10), Gert (August 13–17), Harvey (August 17–31), Irma (August 30-September 12), José (September 5–22), Katia (September 5–9), Lee (September 15–30), Maria (September 16–30), Nate (October 4–9), and Ophelia (October 9–15). Harvey, Irma and Maria were all major hurricanes, meaning they reached Category 3 or higher.

The trio of major hurricanes that crashed into America this year caused what could be the most expensive hurricane season ever, with damage estimates ranging up to $300 to $475 billion. By comparison, the damage from Katrina (2005), which had been the costliest hurricane in US history, was $108 billion.

Franklin was the first of a record-setting streak of ten consecutive hurricanes in the Atlantic Ocean, a feat we have not seen unseen since weather satellites usage starting in the 1960s. (Records for the hurricanes in the Atlantic do go back to the 1800s, but there is a great likelihood that some storms went unnoticed back then.) Only three Category 5 hurricanes have ever made landfall in the US, and 2017 saw two of them (Irma and Maria.) Irma and Maria reached the apex of the scale and made landfall as Category 5 storms. Harvey and José peaked as Category 4 storms. Fueled by warmer water, one storm, Hurricane Ophelia, bizarrely even spiraled as far east as Ireland, the farthest east a hurricane has traveled in modern history.

Hurricane Harvey dumped so much rain over Texas and Louisiana during a week of unending rains that some areas got over four feet of water, the most rainfall amount from a single storm ever recorded in the continental United States.

In the 2017 Atlantic season, Irma was the ninth named storm, the fourth hurricane, the second major hurricane, and the first Category 5 hurricane. Irma was a long and catastrophic hurricane that wreaked havoc over its path and caused calamitous, particularly in the northeastern Caribbean and the Florida Keys.

Only a week later, José and Maria were bearing down on the Caribbean. Maria, a Category 5 hurricane, destroyed the island of Dominica, recovered, and continued with 160-mile per hour winds and made a direct strike on Puerto Rico. Puerto Rico was beaten down by high winds and flooding and resulted in a reported fifty-five deaths (that's the lowest estimate; it could be many times that, according to Puerto Rican officials.) Want to know the site of the largest blackout in US history? Puerto Rico. About 61 percent of the power has been restored but at one time, three to four million people were without power on the island. The cataclysmic damage to Puerto Rico was such that six months later, much of the island has struggled to restore water and power and what was already a tenuous infrastructure is teetering on collapse.

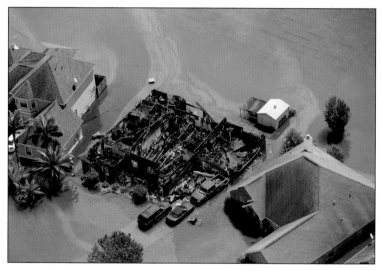

After Hurricane Harvey in Port Arthur, Texas, August 31, 2017.

Harvey and other so-called five-hundred-year floods seem to be happening far more often than that number designation would imply. Some experts are now calling the Harvey floods a thousand-year flood. With all the historic flooding and epic severe weather, we as a society have to ask if these events are really once-in-a-lifetime events? Harvey caused such historic rainfall that entire neighborhoods became submerged. The rainfall totals far exceeded five-hundred-year levels. Harvey was the third storm in three years in Houston to bring so-called five-hundred-year rain to the Bayou City. America has experienced at least twenty-four of these five-hundred-year rain events since 2010.

So what is a five-hundred-year flood? The five-hundred-year term is a risk assessment tool used for flood insurance but does not mean that the event happens only once every five hundred years (like we mistakenly thought). What it does mean is that there is a one in five hundred chance that this amount of flooding will occur in a single year. A hundred-year event has a one in one hundred chance of occurring. What experts tell us is that these large storms and resultant events are happening more often. Why?

This hurricane season brought a warmer Atlantic, and a cooler Pacific. But are we in a new era of hurricanes? Will they continue to be this powerful? Will they become more powerful? Will there be an increase in frequency? Are we prepared? Are you prepared?

Harvey was a potent enough hurricane but it degraded to a tropical cyclone over land. The system spent 117 hours over land, all the while dropping the tremendous amount of rainfall. We have not seen a hurricane, ever, with Irma's brute strength. She held tight to a Category 5 status for three consecutive days while in the Atlantic but even more impressive was that she maintained peak intensity—185 miles per hour—for thirty-seven hours, a world record. Irma smashed into the island of Barbuda in the eastern Caribbean with a direct strike and brought those sustained winds of 185 miles per hour, torrential rain and destructive waves. At least 95 percent of the island's structures—including hospitals, schools, homes and docks—were damaged or destroyed. As of late 2017, the island is virtually de-populated. These are powerful, intense, and record-setting hurricanes. If you believe that our climate continues to warm, that our Atlantic continues to heat up, then it is reasonable to assume that what used to be rare events could even become the norm.

What is a hurricane?

Hurricanes are spiraling, gigantic tropical storms whose wind speeds range from a sustained 74 to 160 miles per hour. Hurricanes gain heat and energy through contact with the warm moist ocean waters. Hurricanes generate "energy" by condensing water vapor and through a process called "heat of condensation." This heat is released into the upper atmosphere....not by precipitation. In fact, hurricanes are like

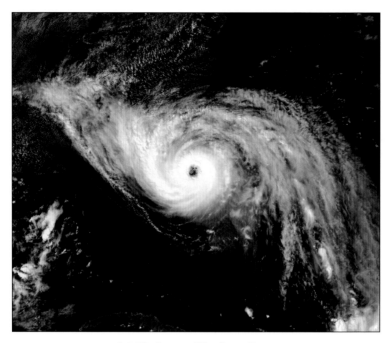

Satellite image of Hurricane Hugo.

ventilation turbines on homes that release attic heat. They take the excess heat from ocean water and release it into the upper atmosphere through the condensation process of making rain.

The center of the storm is called the eye and it is the calmest component, with light winds and fair weather. The eye is surrounded by the eye wall, which is a direct contrast to the calm eye. The eye wall is a violent circle of winds and rain that spiral inward at speeds as high as 200 miles per hour. The entire hurricane can be can be as wide as five hundred to six hundred miles across, while the eye is usually about ten miles across.. In the Northern Hemisphere, hurricanes rotate in a counterclockwise direction around the eye of the storm and in a clockwise direction in the Southern Hemisphere. An Atlantic hurricane usually lasts for a week or more, generally traveling across the ocean at about 10 to 20 miles per hour.

Hurricanes begin over warm ocean water of 80 degrees Fahrenheit or warmer and typically form between 5 to 15 degrees latitude north and south of the equator. The Coriolis force is an inertial energy that acts on objects in motion relative to a rotating reference frame and this force is needed to create the initial spin of the potential hurricane. The spin of the Earth causes objects in the northern hemisphere to turn "to the right." In the Southern Hemisphere, this force causes objects to turn "to the left." For hurricanes, along the Equator and about 5 to 15 degrees north of it, the Coriolis Force is zero or close to it. The Coriolis Force is needed to get that initial group of showers and thunderstorms in the Atlantic or Pacific to start "spinning" and cause a tropical depression to form. The Coriolis force is weakest near the equator, so hurricanes simply never form there. Most hurricanes never make landfall and eventually just peter out harmlessly in the sea.

Some Hurricane Facts

- The Atlantic basin includes the Atlantic Ocean, Caribbean Sea, and Gulf of Mexico. The Eastern Pacific basin extends to 140°W.
- By the beginning of September in an average year we would expect to have had four named systems, two of which would be hurricanes and one of which would be of Category 3 or greater in strength.
- Don't think hurricanes can't hit the northeast; 1954 alone saw three strike the east coast, and in 2012, Superstorm Sandy devastated the Tri-State Area.
- Hurricanes lose strength as they move over land.
- Coastal regions are most at danger from hurricanes but that doesn't mean inland locales can't suffer as the hurricane continues across land.
- In addition to violent winds and heavy rain, hurricanes can also create tornadoes, high waves and widespread flooding.
- Hurricanes are regions of low atmospheric pressure (known as depressions).
- Slow-moving hurricanes produce more rainfall and can cause more damage from flooding than faster-moving, more powerful hurricanes.
- The Atlantic hurricane season is from June 1 to November 30, but most hurricanes occur during the fall months.

The Eastern Pacific hurricane season is from May 15 to November 30.

- The 1970 Bhola Cyclone that struck Bangladesh killed over 300,000 people. In 2005 Hurricane Katrina killed over eighteen hundred people in the United States and caused around $80 billion dollars' worth of property damage. Hurricane Floyd was barely a Category 1 hurricane, but still managed to knock down nearly twenty million trees and caused over a billion dollars in damage.

- Experts estimate that large hurricanes release the energy of ten atomic bombs. Every second. Think about that kind of power for a minute.

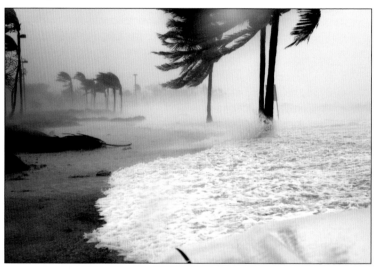

Hurricane winds in Florida. *Credit: Pixabay*

The Spanish mariner-explorers felt the wrath of hurricanes and so the word they gave to these storms was *huracán*, which means evil spirits and weather gods. The same type of storm, a rotating tropical storm with winds at 74 miles per hour or more, has three different names depending on where they originate.

> ➢ **Hurricane** is the name used when these storms develop over the Atlantic or eastern Pacific Oceans.

> ➢ **Cyclones** are the same storms when they form over the Bay of Bengal and the northern Indian Ocean.
> ➢ **Typhoons** are the name for these storms that develop in the western Pacific. (As an extra value added: Australians call hurricanes willy-willies.) The International Date Line is dividing line between the designation of hurricane and tropical storm. Many hurricanes have developed as far West as Hawaii, but become typhoons once they cross the IDL to the west.

The Saffir-Simpson Scale

When a storm's maximum sustained winds reach 74 miles per hour, it is called a hurricane. The National Hurricane Center's official measurement is guided by the Saffir-Simpson Hurricane Wind Scale, which is a 1 to 5 rating, or category, based on a hurricane's maximum sustained winds. The higher the category, the greater the hurricane's potential for property damage. From the wind speed, meteorologists use the Saffir-Simpson Scale to determine the potential damage a hurricane can do. It was first used in hurricane advisories in 1975. Hurricanes are often defined and categorized by their wind speed, but the real danger comes not from furious winds but from the sudden, often fatal rise of the sea or the inundation and subsequent flooding from heavy or continued rains. There is more loss of life through drowning than any other of the various deadly hazards posed by these tropical storms.

Several forces inflict damage on property and life. When a hurricane makes landfall, the storm often produces a devastating storm surge that can reach twenty feet high and extend nearly a hundred miles. The majority of all hurricane deaths are the result of storm surges. The other destructive forces include high winds, tornadoes, torrential rains, and resultant flooding.

Ratings of the Saffir-Simpson Scale

Category 1: 74 to 95 Miles per Hour
- Minimal damage.

- No major damage to properly built structures.
- Damage to unanchored shrubs and trees.
- Evacuations may be ordered for areas immediately adjacent to water.

Category 2: 96 to 100 Miles per Hour
- Moderate damage.
- Some roof, door, and window damage to buildings.
- Considerable damage to shrubs and trees with some trees being blown down.
- Coastal and low lying areas flood two to four hours before arrival of the hurricane's center.
- Evacuations may be ordered for areas near the water.

Category 3: 101 to 130 Miles per Hour
- Extensive damage.
- Structural damage to residences is likely.
- Damage to shrubs and trees with foliage blown off. Large trees are blown down.
- Mobile homes and signs are destroyed.
- Low lying areas flood three to five hours before arrival of the hurricane's center.
- Small structures near coast are destroyed with larger structures being heavily damaged.
- Evacuations will be likely ordered for areas prone to storm-surge flooding.

Category 4: 131 to 155 Miles per Hour
- Extreme damage.
- Complete roofs blown off some residences. Extensive exterior damages to large buildings.
- Shrubs, trees, and all signs are blown down.
- Complete destruction of mobile homes.
- Major damage to lower floors of structures near the store.
- Some coastal buildings may be washed away.
- Evacuations will be likely ordered for areas prone to storm-surge flooding.

Category 5: 155 Miles per Hour or Greater

- Catastrophic damage.
- Complete roof failure on many residences and prefabricated buildings.
- Extensive damage to exposed glass on all large buildings.
- Some complete building failures.
- All shrubs, trees, and signs are blown down.
- Complete destruction of mobile homes.
- Total destruction of all structures near the shoreline.
- Winds from a hurricane can destroy buildings and manufactured homes. Signs, roofing material, and other items left outside can become flying missiles during hurricanes.
- Dangerous waves produced by a tropical cyclone's strong winds can pose a significant hazard to coastal residents and mariners. These waves can cause deadly rip currents, significant beach erosion, and damage to structures along the coastline, even when the storm is more than a thousand miles offshore.

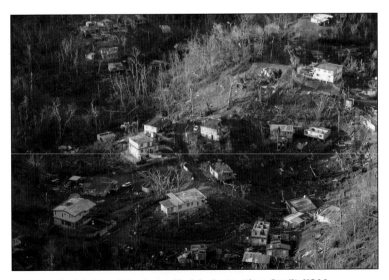

Aerial view of Hurricane Maria's destruction. *Credit: NOAA.*

Hurricane Names

If you're over a certain age, you remember when hurricanes only had female names. Hurricanes now have male and female names. Hurricanes are the only weather disasters that have officially been given their own names. In a weird twist, the first government we know of to provide names to hurricanes? Puerto Rico.

The first hurricane of each year is given a name beginning with the letter "A." In the early 1950s, Atlantic hurricanes identified by the phonetic alphabet, with monikers such as Able-Baker-Charlie. In 1953, the US Weather Bureau made the switch to women's names. Naming rights now go by the World Meteorological Organization, which uses different sets of names that depend on the geographic location of the storm. Until 1979, American hurricanes were only named for women. Since then, the list alternates with men's names too. If a hurricane causes significant damage, that name is retired and replaced with another.

Forces in Hurricanes

Storm surges are almost always the most devastating force of a hurricane. A storm surge occurs when the hurricane's spiraling winds push water forward. When that water hits land, it has nowhere to go as it piles up, so it crashes ashore, sometimes for several miles inland. If you have a storm heading north and you are on the northeast side of the eye of the hurricane, the wind is pushing water toward the shore in advance of the storm, bringing lots of extra water. The lay of the ocean floor nearer the land will influence the rise of storm surge as well. Once you are on the southern side of the storm, the water will recede as it is being pulled away from shore, and will return to normal rather quickly.

So storm surge is water that is the height of the water above the normal tide. Storm surge sometimes reaches as wide as one hundred miles wide and as high as twenty feet high and often brings along with it never-ending, pounding waves.

Storm tide differs from storm surge in that it is the rise in water level during a storm due to the combination of storm surge and the lunar tide. The combination of storm tide with storm surge can bring ashore so much water that the flooding can cause loss of life, destroy homes and buildings, erode beaches, damage roads, and wipe out bridges. Hurricane Katrina (2005) was one of America's most devastating storms in our history. Even though she was a big storm, Katrina was only a Category 3 storm. What made Katrina so deadly was her twenty-eight-foot storm surge. When the hurricane slammed into New Orleans, which sits below sea level, when the levees broke, the city found itself underwater, and around eighteen hundred people lost their lives in the storm, most from drowning. Since most coastal communities on the Atlantic Ocean and Gulf of Mexico are no more than ten feet above sea level, storm surge is the major deadly element of any hurricane that makes landfall.

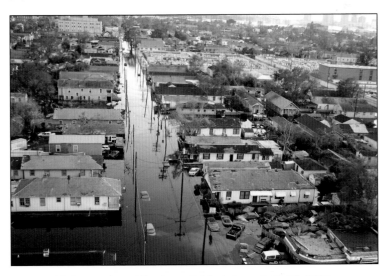

Bird's eye view of Hurricane Katrina's impact. *Credit: NOAA.*

Prediction Models

Think to the times you've watched weather experts on television showing the possible paths of the hurricane heading toward land. The map will have bouncing tennis balls on five to ten differing paths. Some show it will hit directly where you live, some show it turning at the last minute and flailing back out to sea. These predictive models show how difficult and complex it is to properly gauge the route of any hurricane.

Some hurricanes bounce around out at sea, others move turtle-like, and others still surprise all the experts with whopping gains in wind speeds. Every hurricane has its own personality, idiosyncrasies, and potential dangers. Some are simply powerful with less rain but lots of destructive wind (Hurricane Carla, 1961), some are heavy with water (Harvey 2017), some, like Hurricane Andrew (1992), make a direct hit on. Hurricanes move erratically; they zig and zag, diminish and grow, and are often capricious in nature. Every hurricane is different from any other in its unpredictability, growth rates, tracking, and wind to water ratio.

Two models predict hurricane paths, the European model or ECMWF, and the American GFS model. Both models have had histories of success, but in the last few years, they have at times differed greatly in predicting where a hurricane will make landfall. The most notable was Superstorm Sandy. The European model was correct in both the time and area of landfall. The two models are amazingly accurate, all things considered.

If you're interested, you can track each hurricane's path across the ocean, choosing from as many as six apps on your smartphone and several websites. Some of the apps cost a few bucks; some are free.

Types of Hurricanes

- **Tropical Depression:** A tropical cyclone with maximum sustained winds of 38 miles per hour (33 knots) or less.
- **Tropical Storm:** A tropical cyclone with maximum sustained winds of 39 to 73 miles per hour (34 to 63 knots).
- **Hurricane:** A tropical cyclone with maximum sustained winds of 74 miles per hour (64 knots) or

higher. In the western North Pacific, hurricanes are called typhoons; similar storms in the Indian Ocean and South Pacific Ocean are called cyclones.

• **Major Hurricane:** A tropical cyclone with maximum sustained winds of 111 miles per hour (96 knots) or higher, corresponding to a Category 3, 4, or 5 on the Saffir-Simpson Hurricane Wind Scale.

Hurricane Levels

➢ **Tropical Storm Watch:** Tropical Storm conditions with sustained winds from 39 to 74 miles per hour are possible in your area within the next thirty-six hours.

➢ **Tropical Storm Warning:** Tropical Storm conditions are expected in your area within the next twenty-four hours.

➢ **Hurricane Watch:** Hurricane conditions with sustained winds of 74 miles per hour or greater are possible in your area within the next thirty-six hours. This watch should trigger your family's disaster plan, and protective measures should be initiated. If you need to leave the area, secure a boat, or exit an island, this is the time to do so.

➢ **Hurricane Warning:** Hurricane conditions are expected in your area within twenty-four hours. Once this warning has been issued, your family should be in the process of completing emergency actions and deciding the safest location to be during the storm.

➢ **Coastal Flood Watch:** The possibility exists for the inundation of land areas along the coast within the next twelve to thirty-six hours.

➢ **Coastal Flood Warning:** Land areas along the coast are expected to become, or have become, inundated by seawater above the typical tide action.

➢ **Small Craft Advisory:** A small craft advisory is a type of warning issued by the National Weather Service, most frequently in coastal areas. It is issued when winds have reached, or are expected to reach within twelve hours, a speed marginally less than that which is considered gale force, usually 25 to 38 miles per hour.

Hurricanes are of course the biggest threat to property and life, but don't overlook the devastation that tropical storms or tropical depressions can bring. These lesser storms can still cause storm surge flooding, inland flooding from heavy rains, destructive winds, tornadoes, and high surf and rip currents.

We have to add a quick note about a cyclone we'd never, ever heard about before, the 2018 bomb cyclone. A monster storm has developed off the eastern seaboard and will hammer coastal locations all along the western Atlantic and US East Coast with ice, snow, and high winds—in essence, a winter hurricane. Meteorologists called this event a bomb cyclone because its pressure is predicted to fall rapidly, a marker of explosive strengthening and typical of hurricanes—a low pressure rotating storm system with winds as high as 74 miles per hour. In winter! Blizzard conditions were reached quickly. The storm was big and powerful and had a gigantic circulation that pulled in the polar vortex, that frigid air zone that circles the North Pole.

Preparation

Hurricanes are the weather disasters that provide the longest lead time in terms of preparation. So you have plenty of time to get ready. No excuses. So ask yourself—do you live in a storm surge and hurricane evacuation zone? If so, you need to prepare. If you live in the South within a couple of hours of the coast, prepare. If you live on the East Coast, prepare. If you live in the Caribbean, well, you really need to prepare.

Warning fatigue is a major problem for community safety. If you are advised to leave but you stay anyway, and things get rough, some emergency personnel might have to get out in the thick of bad weather to rescue you. Warning fatigue is the affliction that occurs to people who choose, against information, expertise, and common sense, to ignore the experts' warnings. Warning fatigue, or hurricane fatigue, is when you say out loud "hurricanes have been predicted to hit but passed by us before" or a "hurricane hit before and it wasn't as bad as they said or we are tough, so let's drink and bring in the hurricane," etc. Just because you haven't felt the entire wrath of a hurricane before, doesn't mean that this time it won't put you and your property in much worse danger.

The time to prepare for a hurricane is before the season begins, when you have the time and are not under pressure. If you wait until a hurricane is pounding the beaches near your house, you've waited too late and you put your family and property in danger. Start preparing for an eventual hurricane by making your home more hurricane-resistant, creating an emergency management plan, and prepare by putting together supplies, a hurricane getaway bag, house survival kit.

Atlantic hurricane season begins on June 1 and officially ends November 30 although hurricanes have been known to happen well into December. You'll want to prepare your home and survival kit well before that date. You need to understand your home's vulnerability to storm surge, flooding, and wind. Trim limbs and remove damaged trees near your house because hurricane winds can knock them down and damage your property. Tighten up any loose rain gutters and downspouts. Remove any clogged areas or debris to prevent backflooding and water damage to your property. Install hurricane window shutters. Retrofit your windows and doors, your garage doors, and your roof. If you are really serious about hurricane safety, and have the extra money, think about building an above-flood-level FEMA safe room storm shelter designed for protection from high winds. If you can afford it, you can install plywood hurricane shutters.

If you own a boat, you won't want to leave it tied up at the dock. Decide where to move your vessel if the hurricane is headed your way. Review your insurance policy and add flood coverage if you can. Take videos or photos of your property because it's easier and more complete than taking inventory on a notepad. And make sure you have insurance on that boat.

Planning

Sit down with your family members and take the time now to write down your hurricane plan. Think about the possible places you would stay during a hurricane, under what circumstances you would leave (short of an evacuation demand), and what supplies you will need. Decide how you will get in contact with each other, where you will go, and what you will do to make sure you are all safe in an emergency. Keep a copy of this plan as a document in your computer and cloud, as a paper copy in your emergency supplies kit, with each person in your house and in another safe place where you can access it in the event of a hurricane and/or flood.

Determine safe evacuation routes moving inland and have second and third options if hotels fill up along the way. Learn the locations of official shelters. Make emergency plans for pets. Coordinate where to meet up if you won't be in the same place or same car when you leave. Determine whom each of you will contact to let the others know you are safe.

You need to check your home and determine its vulnerability to storm surge, flooding, and wind. You need to know your surroundings and learn your community hurricane evacuation routes and how to find and get to higher ground. Write down or print out emergency contacts, keep them handy, and also put them in every family member's smartphone. It's a great idea, albeit difficult to get motivation to do so, but your family should take first-aid, CPR, and disaster-preparedness classes.

Since the supplies you really need will be gone by the time you can run to the grocery store or building supply house, it makes sense to buy some of these and store them ahead of time. If a hurricane gets mentioned on the news as possibly heading your way, count on gas shortages, traffic on major highways, as well as a run on groceries, plywood, generators, and water. Sometimes you can find plywood and other supplies at distribution centers but it'll be crowded. So you need to have a ready supply of essentials beforehand. If you are prepared before a hurricane heads for your home, you have made the odds in your favor that you will be a successful hurricane survivor.

You need to check your home and determine the vulnerability to storm, surge, flooding and wind. You need to know your surroundings and learn your community hurricane evacuation routes and how to find and get to higher ground. You and your family should plan escape routes from your home, but most importantly places to meet.

Call your insurance agent and ask for an insurance checkup. You want to ensure you have enough homeowners' insurance to repair or replace your home, if necessary. Don't forget coverage for your car or boat. Since standard homeowners' insurance doesn't cover flooding, you'll need a separate policy for it, and it should be available through your agent or the National Flood Insurance Program at www.floodsmart.gov. Act now as flood insurance requires a thirty-day waiting period.

Have plywood in your shed so you can board up windows and doors in case of an emergency. In high winds trees and shrubs can be lifted up, so rid yourself of any rotted ones, and trim your trees and shrubs from iffy limbs so you will have less tree debris in your yard after the storm.

Learn the elevation level and flood risk of your property. Make sure you have cleared loose and clogged rain gutters and downspouts so you don't create a water drainage problem for yourself. If your area floods frequently, your local hardware stores probably sell empty bags for DIY sandbags. Stack the bags on a waterproof tarp to create a barrier against mild flooding.

Supplies

Redundancy is good in this case. Having two of everything is a good idea. In case one goes out, breaks, doesn't work, or gets wet, having a backup is sensible. So where do you even start?

Start with food and water. Buy food that will keep and buy lots of drinking water in bottles and jugs. You may need to survive on your own after an emergency. This means having your own food, water, and other supplies in sufficient quantity to last for at least seventy-two hours, maybe more. You're going to need supplies; not just to get through the storm but for the potentially lengthy and unpleasant aftermath. Have enough non-perishable food, water, and medicine to last each person in your family a minimum of one week. Electricity and water could be out for at least that long. Check emergency equipment, such as flashlights, generators, and storm shutters.

- Drinking water. At a minimum, have enough for three days. If you can, store enough water for three weeks. Also, if you get stranded and have to find alternative water sources, have iodine tablets or a filtration system (backpacker style) on hand.
- Canned and dry food. You might investigate backpacker food—just add boiling water.
- Propane camp stove. (You probably won't have electricity.)
- Generator and gasoline. If the power goes out, and the chances are good it will, you can keep the power with a generator. See a professional about what generator best meets your needs.
- Battery-operated weather radio; or even better, a secondary hand-crank radio in case the batteries lose charge.
- Portable alarm clock.
- Manual can opener.
- Paper plates, plastic ware, or metal eating utensils.
- Extra batteries.
- Trash bags.
- Flashlights. You need several, including a head lamp.
- Extension cords.
- Rope or nylon cord.
- Waders. Simply buy some chest waders, like those that hunters and anglers use.
- Map of the area, including an agreed-upon meeting spot in case of separation and the nearest safe shelter.
- Shoes. We're fisherman and have used lightweight sandals designed for wading. They are lightweight, have grip, and are ideal for the kit. Flip-flops won't work in flood

conditions—they will come off, leaving your feet exposed to underwater dangers, but shoes designed for wading will keep you better protected. A pair of old canvas slip-on tennis shoes with a thick rubber sole would work too.

- Rain gear.
- Duct tape.
- Sleeping bags and pillows.
- Blankets.
- Tarp.
- Mosquito repellant.
- Candles.
- Matches, lighters.
- Water jugs and water purification tablets.
- Change or two of clothes, underwear, rain jacket, sturdy flat shoes.
- Prescription medicine, pain reliever, antibiotic, anti-diarrhea, etc.
- First-aid kit. You can use one you purchase off the shelf but if you do, add more to it that fits your needs.
- Cash and change, as ATMs and banks probably won't be working.
- A sheet and markers to make banners for a roof sign.

Tools for after the storm, including:

➢ Hammer and nails
➢ Shovel
➢ Hand saw
➢ Broom
➢ Screwdrivers
➢ Crescent wrench
➢ Pipe wrench
➢ Pliers
➢ Limb Saw
➢ Utility knife

- ➢ Machete
- ➢ Vise Grips
- ➢ Work Gloves
- ➢ A couple of sheets of plywood, preferably 2x4s, in case you need to leave the house and not leave it open to vandalism or looting
- ➢ Ziplock bags of all sizes because it'll be wet everywhere and you don't want your phone getting fried. Put your important papers in ziplock baggies.
- ➢ Power backups such as a generator. You may not have either electricity or cell phone service for a while. Use all safety procedures for generators. Have written instructions for turning off.
- ➢ Pet food, bowls for water and food, medicines they need, and leash. If you have to take them with you, make sure the motels or the hotels from your list are pet friendly.

Additionally, have a basic grab-n-go bag ready for each family member: It should include clothes, sleeping gear (if you plan to go to a temporary shelter or stay in a hotel/motel out of harm's way), food and water, and some form of leisure (small board game, a book, or the like.)

Smartphones

The smartphones in your family are probably your second most important resource (behind food/water). Keep them dry by using waterproof phones, waterproof cases, or ziplock baggies. Carry your chargers with you but consider adding a portable battery pack. You can often get an hour or two extra charge out of these. One great battery booster for your phone is a hand-crank booster; there several models available online. If you have your vehicle during the hurricane event, you can plug your devices into your car's cigarette lighter.

You might not know that you do not need to have an active phone plan to call 911 from any smartphone. If you have cell service, send out text messages and emails, and post notifications to Facebook and Twitter about your whereabouts and immediate needs. Facebook Check-In has proven easy and useful in emergencies. In the event you have power and Wi-Fi, but no cellular, there are apps that let you make video and audio calls for help. By using apps like Facebook Messenger, Google Duo, Viber, and others, you can still make free phone calls over Wi-Fi even if there's no cell service. Some may require you setting this up ahead of time. Skype is also free to another Skype user.

Download maps to access offline. This way, your mapping function will still work on your smartphone just like the old standalone GPS navigation units. You are limited and the smartphone is less accurate, won't have real time traffic or info, but it can still help you get from point A to point B without cell service through the GPS sensor.

When a hurricane threatens your home and community, be prepared to evacuate. Allow enough time to pack and inform friends and family if you need to leave your home. You do have a week to prepare—boarding up the house, moving stuff up to highest point or putting in storage, gassing up car, having survival kits in the car or house, having a plan, batteries and radio, common sense and listening to authorities, escape routes, boats, and waders.

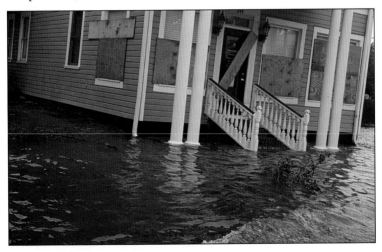

Boarded windows during Hurricane Matthew. *Credit: USDA of Edisto Beach, Edisto Island, South Carolina.*

Cover all of your home's windows. Permanent storm shutters offer the best protection for windows. A second option is to board up windows with 5/8-inch exterior grade or marine plywood. Experts say that taping your windows in preparation for a hurricane is a waste of time and money. Tape does not strengthen glass at all and debris will smash a taped window as if the tape wasn't there.

Check the websites of your local National Weather Service office and local government/emergency management office. Find out what type of emergencies could occur and how you should respond. Listen to NOAA Weather Radio or other radio or TV stations for the latest storm news. Follow instructions issued by local officials. Leave immediately if ordered.

Survival

Most folks have at one point in their lives witnessed wind gusts exceeding 70 miles per hour, perhaps even 80 miles per hour. But when winds gusting to nearly 140 miles per hour are expected, how can we compare? An important thing to note is that there is an exponential increase in damage and force as speed ticks up. In other words, 140 mile per hour winds won't be twice as strong, but rather four times as strong as winds of 70 miles per hour.

If you're safe from surge but find yourself facing extreme winds, seek shelter in the most interior room on the lowest floor of your home or business, and avoid windows; a basement would be preferable. This only applies to site-built homes. Outbuildings, mobile homes, vehicles, and any other unanchored structures will not suffice, and the consequences could be deadly. Mobile homes will disintegrate in extreme winds, with shrapnel acting as lethal projectiles, jeopardizing the lives of anyone nearby.

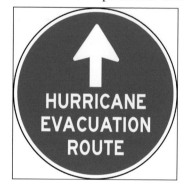

Hurricane watch = conditions possible within the next forty-eight hours.

Steps to take:

- Review your evacuation route(s) and listen to local officials.
- Review the items in your disaster supply kit and add items to meet the household needs for children, parents, individuals with disabilities or other access and functional needs, and pets.

Hurricane warning = conditions are expected within thirty-six hours.

- Follow evacuation orders from local officials, if given.
- Check in with family and friends by texting or using social media.
- Follow the hurricane timeline preparedness checklist, depending on when the storm is anticipated to hit and the impact that is projected for your location.

What to do when a hurricane is one to six hours from arriving:

- If you have not been ordered to evacuate, stay at home, and let friends and family know where you are.
- Last minute boarding of windows, positioning of sand bags. If you installed storm shutters, shut them and stay away from windows.
- Turn your refrigerator or freezer to the coldest setting and open only when necessary. Freeze jugs of water and leave them in the freezer to maintain cold if the power goes off. If you have a thermometer to check fridge and freezer temperature, have it handy. You don't want to eat spoiled food.
- Turn on your television and your NOAA. Go back and forth between the Weather Channel and your local stations. Check your city/county website every thirty minutes in order to get the latest weather updates and emergency instructions.
- Revisit your supplies, move valuables to a higher floor or place them in watertight tubs or bags, fill up the tub with

water, get into survival mode. Use water in bathtubs for cleaning and flushing only. Do NOT drink it.
- Turn off propane tanks. Unplug small appliances.

What to do when a hurricane is six to eighteen hours from arriving
- Maintain ongoing awareness with your TV/radio, checking your city or county website every thirty minutes in order to get the latest weather updates and emergency instructions.
- Have a meeting with family and revisit evacuation and emergency plans.
- Charge your cell phones so you will have a full battery in case you lose power.

What to do when a hurricane is eighteen to thirty hours from arriving
- Pull up your city or county website for quick access to storm updates and emergency instructions.
- Remove lightweight objects outside and inside that could become missiles in high winds such as (e.g., patio furniture, folding chairs, trash cans.)
- Cover all of your home's windows with plywood. Screws rather than nails. If you have permanent storm shutters, close them and cover your windows. A second option is to board up windows with 5/8-inch exterior grade or marine plywood, cut to fit and ready to install.

What to do when a hurricane is three days or more from arriving
- Turn on your TV and radio to get the latest weather updates and emergency instructions.
- Build or restock your emergency preparedness kit. You might stand in some lines but you're still three days out so it might not be too bad. Include food and water sufficient for at least seventy-two hours or more, medicine, flashlights, batteries, cash, and first-aid supplies.
- If you have not put together an emergency plan, do it now. Sit down with everyone in your household and plan how to

communicate with each if you lose power or are in different places in town. Review your evacuation plan with your family. You may have to leave quickly so plan ahead.
- Fill your gas tank, stock your vehicle with emergency supplies, and have your grab bags handy.

If there is an evacuation order for your region, don't consider being one of the crazies you see on the news who stay despite all warnings. Sometimes you'll see these locals who are at the beach bar drinking Mai Tais at a hurricane party and celebrating their lunacy of beating back the storm. If the experts have determined your community should evacuate, then evacuate. If you stay, you not only put yourself in danger, but also first responders who have to come save you. Some people won't or can't leave even if an evacuation order is given. Some can't get out due to disabilities. Others aren't locked into monitoring social media and rarely watch the news so they just don't know the severe risk.

Some people don't want to board their pets or feel they can't take them with them (we all have that aunt with sixteen cats), so they are reluctant to leave their pets behind. Some won't leave from fear of their home being damaged or thieves looting their property. Some who won't leave remember the last few hurricane warnings and how they weathered the storm successfully.

If your home is close to sea level or in a flood-prone location, leave early to minimize the risk of getting stuck in traffic or missing the window of safely exiting. As you travel during evacuation, know that you will likely encounter heavy traffic. Go slow, drive smart, and monitor the news.

If you are forced to remain, storm safety rules are the same: Remain inside a secure shelter and stay away from windows. Even when it seems like the hurricane has calmed, stay in a safe place; you could simply be in the eye of the storm, which provides a brief lull. Make sure you learn the location of shelters in your area in advance.

Plan to evacuate if you live in a mobile or manufactured home. These types of unstable construction are simply unsafe in high winds no matter if fastened to the ground or not. Evacuate if you live right on a coastline, on an offshore island, or near a river or floodplain. You will be enduring not only high winds, but flooding from storm surge waves and other flooding. Evacuate if you live in a high-rise. Hurricane winds can knock out electricity to elevators and break windows. The winds are worse the higher you go.

You'll see this posted on Facebook every disaster and it rings true, ought to be true, but it's not: The gist of the fake news is that hotels must accommodate pets belonging to evacuees and if they claim otherwise, call FEMA or threaten them with FEMA. It's just not true. Hotels must only accept service animals. They are not required to take in pets, so evacuees with pets should check hotel policy. Some hotels and motels do accept pets but most don't. Emergency shelters are required to take both the pets and service animals of evacuees.

So you are in the midst of evacuating. Stay alert to storm advisories by using your NOAA weather radio. Enact your family emergency plan. Map out your route using travel routes specified by local authorities. Bring your grab-n-go kits. Make sure you included your important documents. In the trunk, store enough food and water for at three days, just in case you get stranded or there's a shortage where you are going. Notify your family and friends of your plans.

If You're Not Evacuating

When the hurricane is an hour or two away.

- Blow out candles or any other open flames (fireplace).
- Use the stairs, not the elevator.
- Alert your emergency contacts and family/friends of your status.
- Stay away from unprotected windows. It's going to be hard not to take periodic peeks out your window to see what's going on but don't do it. The wind speeds can gust and break out windows.
- Check your fridge and re-locate any food you're planning on eating during the storm to coolers with ice.

- Think about which trees in your yard may fall and what part of the house they would crush. Don't situate yourself there.
- Closely monitor radio, TV, or NOAA Weather Radio.
- Close storm shutters.

If you're riding out the storm in a high rise, it is especially important that you stay away from the windows. If something flies off a neighboring building, it can smash windows downwind. Besides that, the wind is stronger because you're higher in the air, and the air gets squeezed between the tall buildings. The high wind stresses the glass, and makes it break more violently if something hits it.

The hurricane is upon you:
- Stay away from low-lying and flood-prone areas.
- Take shelter in a small interior room, closet, or hallway on the lowest level during the storm. Put as many walls between you and the outside as you can.
- Stay low wherever you are.
- Always stay indoors during a hurricane, because strong winds blow loose items around. If you go outside, you put yourself in harm's way.
- If you have a basement, get there quickly. But if you don't have a basement? The advice still holds: get as low to the ground as you can, in the lowest part of your house. After the worst passes and you see flooding in the basement, get back up to ground level.
- If you can tell things outside are getting bad, go to a central bathroom, drag a mattress inside, and use it to cover yourself and any family members. Bathrooms are usually the most stable rooms due to the complex web of pipework woven into the walls.
- Use a mattress as an extra line of defense no matter where you are in your house.
- Stay away from windows, skylights, and glass doors.

- If the eye of the storm passes over your area, there will be a short period of calm, but at the other side of the eye, the wind speed rapidly increases to hurricane force winds coming from the opposite direction.
- If this is a slow-moving hurricane, you might be riding this out for as much as six to twelve hours so get comfortable and safe.

Aftermath

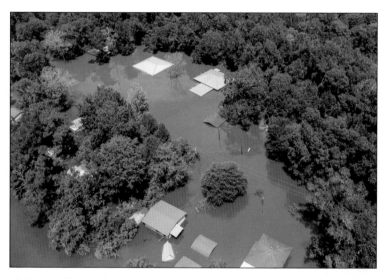

Submerged homes in Port Arthur, Texas. *Credit: South Carolina National Guard.*

The hurricane might have taken a last-minute turn and missed your community entirely. But don't get too excited because you're not out of the woods yet. Tornadoes often form in the front-right quadrant of a hurricane as the storm hits land and decays, tornadoes are spawned. They are often numerous but usually less powerful than your normal tornado. Because they come from less powerful cells, they are less observable on radar, less predictable, and have much less thunder and lightning than normal storms. Nevertheless, these brief but plentiful tornadoes can do damage even though the worst of the hurricane seems over.

A storm surge could have left standing water that has flooded homes, caused creeks to swell, and forced evacuations. Winds could have damaged trees and utility poles, impaled objects through into your house, damaged your car, broken windows in buildings, and so much more.

The most dangerous post-landfall force of any hurricane are the heavy rains that deluge any community in its landward path. Hurricane Harvey's main force hit well south of Houston but set up in a whirling constant deluge as it moved slowly east and up the Texas Coast, especially over the Houston area.

Harvey's flooding resulted in one of the worst weather disasters in US history; the cost will amount to billions of dollars. An estimated 70 percent of Harris County, Texas was flooded by at least 1.5 feet of water. There was an estimated 136,000 flooded structures in the county alone.

The top rainfall total from Harvey was a record-setting 60.58 inches in Nederland, Texas over a period from August 24 to September 1. Groves, Texas, also received more than sixty inches during that same time period. Both of these amounts topped the previous tropical hurricane rainfall record. This rainfall total was more than the forty-eight-inch storm total in Medina, Texas, from Tropical Storm Amelia in 1978.

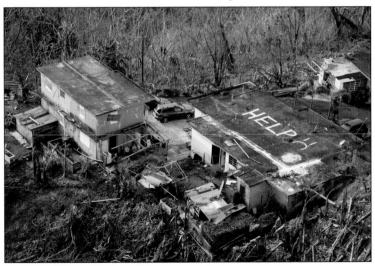

Rooftop SOS, Puerto Rico, 2017. *Credit: US Customs and Border Protection.*

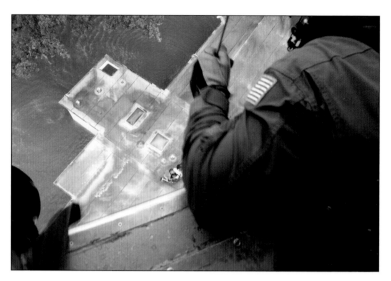

A roof rescue during Hurricane Harvey.
Credit: Petty Officer 3rd Class Johanna Strickland, US Coast Guard.

What can happen after the hurricane passes? Flooding, power loss, refrigeration loss, lack of cell service, no food or clean water, no gasoline, blocked roads, destroyed airplane runways, interrupted city infrastructure, police and fire overload, no access to medical help can all happen. And that's not all of it.

So the aftermath of hurricanes can be as deadly as the main thrust. The hurricane you just survived could have ended up being much worse than you thought; might've surpassed the critical prognostications of the weather experts. So now what?

Think of Katrina in New Orleans, Harvey in Houston, and Irma in Puerto Rico. Think of how flooded things were—houses underwater, water so deep on freeways that the water nearly touched the big green off-ramp signs, bayous swollen like huge lakes. Remember how Puerto Rico and the Virgin Islands after Irma and Maria looked like war zones in the aftermath. FEMA, the National Guard, and Red Cross were there after each hurricane on the mainland and on the islands to provide aid but what stands out were the citizens in action, those in their own boats rescuing those in peril, those wading through chest-deep water to save a dog, locate victims held hostage by the storm. Many responders came from all parts of the country. It was rewarding to witness so many risking their lives for others.

If a hurricane plows through a community, it becomes a survival endeavor, and each time, the community steps up. Many individuals take food and water to stranded victims, cooking for them and providing shelter. Churches also step up and are often instrumental in aftermath safety. If it happens to you, you may want to be a responder. If the worst has happened and your community got hit by high winds or terrible flooding and government and service charities are overwhelmed and cannot fully help, you may want to be part of the solution. The best advice is not to wait until the hurricane hits, but get involved with your community and its emergency planning beforehand.

Thousands of water rescues occurred in the Houston metro area as many homes and businesses were swamped by floodwaters. People were stranded on the roofs of their homes. Storm surges and heavy rain can cause such terrible flooding that you may be driven to your roof. Here's a key—be ready for it. Have the tools to cut out or knock out or axe out a passage to roof. Have supplies stored (waterproofed) up in the attic. Food and water are the two main resources to have for survival in the attic or on the roof. First responders need to find you. How can you help them help you? Do you have some way to signal them?

Some victims eventually decide they need to leave the roof for various reasons. They often use taped-up coolers, life vests, or even pool floaties to get away. If you do this, watch for submerged dangers and take a waterproofed survival kit.

The danger has passed, you might think, but it's only just beginning. The inundation of water will drive snakes to find dry space which means they may be swimming in the water in which you are wading, or finding dry shelter in your house. One of the dangers in the Harvey aftermath were swarms of fire ants pushed out by the waters. Flood water is often contaminated with chemicals, sewage, and other contaminants. You may find road closures and detours, power outages, no running water, unstable houses and buildings, degraded bridges and roads, gas leaks, and looting. Yes, looting does happen after disasters when a handful of people take advantage of the vulnerability of a community but it's overrated. The Houston area only had two hundred arrests after Harvey but this was in a city with five-plus million people. So yes, be worried about looting, but not overly so.

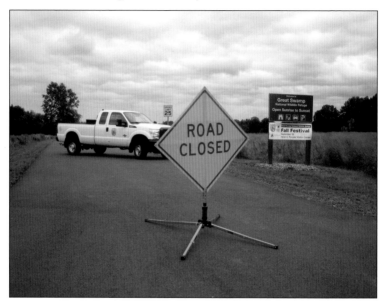

Observe road closures. *Credit: US Fish and Wildlife Service.*

Watch for closed roads. If you come upon a barricade or a flooded road, then turn around, don't drown! Avoid weakened bridges and washed out roads. Stay on firm ground. If the water is moving, don't wade through it. Moving water only six inches deep can sweep you off your feet. Watch out for flooding, which can happen after a hurricane. Stay away from standing water. It may be electrically charged from underground or downed power lines. The chapter on floods in this book has great advice on how to deal with post-hurricane flooding.

As you wade through murky water, submerged dangers exist that can cut and stick you. E-coli can be present in dirty floodwater. Simply, buy some chest waders. You may have to help neighbors, become a first responder, go out for food, supplies, or medicine, or move from your house to shelter. Stay dry while keeping your legs and feet safe from cuts and contaminated water. If you have to wade, there are dangers—snakes and other animals, chemicals and sewage in floodwater, sharp objects underwater, electrical cables, and water that can sweep you away or trap you underneath.

Obtaining fresh water and food, as well as medicine and medical attention, will be difficult to impossible. Cell service may be interrupted, so even locating open shelters or paths out to safety may not be an option. You may be on your own for a good bit. If you evacuated, you may not be able to get back home for a few days, a week, or depending on the damage, much longer. And when you do get back, what will you find?

Once home, check gas, water, and electrical lines and appliances for damage. Use a flashlight to inspect for damage. Never use candles and other open flames indoors. Do not drink or prepare food with tap water until officials give the thumbs up. Stay indoors until it is safe to come out. Check for injured or trapped people, without putting yourself in danger.

- Listen to local officials for updates and instructions.
- Check-in with family and friends by texting or using social media.
- Return home only when authorities indicate it is safe.
- Watch out for debris and downed power lines.
- Avoid walking or driving through floodwaters. Just six inches of moving water can knock you down, and one foot of fast-moving water can sweep your vehicle away.
- Avoid floodwater as it may be electrically charged from underground or downed power lines and may hide dangerous debris or places where the ground is washed away.
- Photograph the damage to your property in order to assist in filing an insurance claim.
- Do what you can to prevent further damage to your property (e.g., putting a tarp on a damaged roof), as insurance may not cover additional damage that occurs after the storm.

- Continue listening to a NOAA Weather Radio or the local news for the latest updates. If you have evacuated, return home only when officials say it is safe.
- Once home, drive only if necessary and avoid flooded roads and washed-out bridges. If you must go out, watch for fallen objects in the road, downed electrical wires, and weakened walls, bridges, roads, and sidewalks that might collapse.
- Walk carefully around the outside of your home to check for loose power lines, gas leaks, and structural damage.
- Stay out of any building if you smell gas, if floodwaters remain around the building, if the building or home was damaged by fire, or if the authorities have not declared it safe.
- Carbon monoxide poisoning is one of the leading causes of death after storms in areas dealing with power outages. Never use a portable generator inside your home or garage.
- Use battery-powered flashlights. Do not use candles. Turn on your flashlight before entering a vacated building. The battery could produce a spark that could ignite leaking gas, if present.

If you have to go to a shelter:

You will encounter a true picture of who comprises your community, mingle with an intimate collection of all kinds of people from your town, folks from all walks of life, all kinds of hygiene choices, sleeping arrangements, and clothing options. It can feel intimidating and weird. But you have no choice, so make the best of it. You and your family are no more (or no less) important than anyone else in the shelter.

Follow the rules. You are in public, with others who have volunteered their time to help out hundreds or thousands. This is not the volunteer's full-time job, they're not getting paid and they're doing the best they can. This is no time to be rebellious. Fit in. Help out. Help with the trash, help an older person, or comfort someone crying. Observe lights-out time. This is a stressful situation so don't make it more stressful for them.

Take only the minimum with you. Whatever can fit into a small backpack or bag. No alcohol, cigarettes or vapes, or illegal drugs. The shelter will be basic, likely a gym or auditorium; it will probably be crowded, and definitely nothing fancy. Be on good behavior. Don't cuss and don't talk about politics or religion. Be aware if you are a loud-talker (non-whisperer) that your voice may carry. Be self-aware.

Don't bring any guns. Period. But a pocketknife? Your call. We would. We wouldn't flash it, wouldn't pull it out to show any aggressive behavior but, hey, you might need it for practical utility reasons anyway.

Bring your own pillow and sheets if you can, but if not, stay dressed at all times, and sleep in your clothes too. You can fit a small throw blanket in your backpack to use. You don't want to have to worry about changing into pajamas and back again. Just sleep in loose-fitting warm clothes that can wrinkle.

Don't forget medicine and hygiene items. You don't know how long you are going to be at the shelter, so bring enough for a week at least. Bring your own toothbrush, soap, toothpaste, deodorant, towels, diapers, and washrag.

Take care of your pets. If you're at a pet-friendly shelter, make sure your pets are supervised, are on a leash, and don't intrude on others. Bring their food and medicine, toys and leashes.

Things could get boring. Be ready to entertain yourself and your family. Bring toys, books, magazines, crosswords, iPad, and your cellphone. Remember that if you are showy with snacks or games, others may see and invade your privacy and ask, "You don't happen to have an extra Coke? Can I see that magazine after you?" Show compassion, but perhaps be less showy too.

The bathroom and shower situations can be tricky. You may be faced with a group shower. Depending on how funky you smell, we recommend not taking a shower for a day or two until you get a vibe on how the shower cycle works and how much privacy you can be afforded. The toilets will hopefully be private, but they may not be. You may have to deal with lower water pressure and lots of people using the facilities. You shouldn't use your normal toilet time habits either. Get in and get out. Use hand wipes to clean the toilet seat and your hands. Toilet paper is at a premium in public toilets and it's often thin and cheap. Bring your own.

<u>What to Bring to the Shelter</u>

- Flashlights, one per person
- Extra batteries
- A blanket or sleeping bag for each person
- Identification
- Valuable papers such as insurance policies
- Cash and credit card
- First aid kit
- Medicine
- Sanitary hand gel
- Baby food and diapers
- Cards, games, books, music players with headphones
- Toiletries, hand wipes, and a roll of toilet paper
- Battery-powered radio, cell phone, and charger
- Snacks

Emergency and damage assessment officials generally make the first survey of land areas affected by the hurricane in order to identify priority areas for cleanup. They will determine a financial loss evaluation which in turn determines the need for a disaster declaration. If the local government is unable to financially recover from the destruction caused by a hurricane, state and/or federal government officials will request an "official" declaration. Once declared as an official disaster, additional state and federal agencies will come to the aid of local government.

Clean-up and recovery operations will begin in the following priority:

1. Search and rescue for disaster victims
2. Clear roadways used by emergency vehicles. Ensure the integrity of the water systems
3. Restore sewer systems operations
4. Restore communications

5. Restore power
6. Remove debris

All clean-up and recovery activities will be coordinated with other assisting agencies and utility companies.

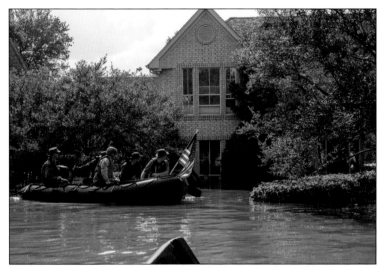

Boat rescue in Houston after Hurricane Harvey.
Credit: Lance Corporal Niles Lee, US Marine Corps.

Returning Home

Discover if local authorities have declared your neighborhood safe. Officials may close certain roads due to flooding or suspected road damage but as you drive, keep an eye out for road hazards like debris and sinkholes. Authorities may have established specific routes so follow those. It's a good idea to return home during daylight hours so you won't need to turn on the lights. Stay in touch with family and friends. Alert others of your status and plans to return home. Remain aware. Keep your radio tuned to local news and emergency broadcasts for updated information. Check the apps and text alerts.

Do not drive through any water. You don't know what's under the water and standing water might be hiding large sinkholes or road damage. You might stall your vehicle if it's deeper than you estimated which puts you in a more dangerous situation.

Be aware of fallen electrical power lines. Do not drive over them or through any water that may contain downed lines. If power lines fall upon your vehicle while driving, continue to drive away from the danger. Wait for emergency rescue personnel and warn other bystanders away from your vehicle and potential danger.

Just because buildings and homes look undamaged does not mean that they don't have hidden dangers of flood damage. Don't work in or around any building until it has been examined and certified safe by professional engineers or architects. Leave the area immediately if you feel the building shifting or if you hear unusual noises that may signal a possible collapse.

Don't turn on any lights, smoke, light matches, or do anything that could cause a spark. Do not return to your house until you are told it is safe to do so. Do you smell gas? If you smell gas or suspect a leak, turn off the main valve, open the windows, and leave the building immediately. Alert your local gas company, as well as local police and fire departments.

If you see frayed wiring, sparks from wires, or smell something burning but see no evidence of fire, you may have electrical damage. You need to shut off the electric system at your home's main circuit breaker or fuse box.

Clean up Safely

Wear proper protective clothing before you get started cleaning up your house. Put on heavy-duty work gloves, sturdy shoes or boots, a long-sleeved shirt, and thick pants. Think about wearing a hard hat because things could fall upon your head and potentially cause a concussion.

Be cautious of contamination and chemicals. Floodwaters and high winds may have put things into the soil or the water. Be alert for animal dangers. Wild or stray domestic pets will be disoriented just like humans after a natural disaster. Wild animals like snakes, alligators, or rats can be in your yard or house because they were driven there by high water. As you pick up debris from piles, know that these are

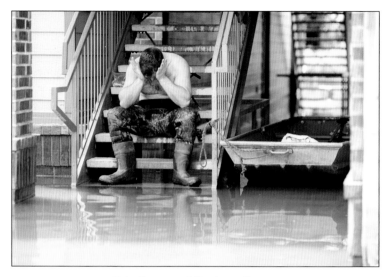

Katy, Texas, post-Hurricane Harvey.

hiding places for these kinds of animals. Call your local Animal Control office to deal with strays and disoriented pets. Contact Animal Control authorities for information on how to dispose of dead animals found on your property.

Don't wade into the water if you aren't wearing chest waders. Standing floodwater on your property may hide a host of dangers including live electrical lines and fecal matter from overflowed sewage lines. Do not let children play in any water or touch objects that may have been exposed to possibly contaminated water. Be prepared for fire hazards. Always have at least two fire extinguishers at the cleanup site.

Beware of spoiled food. Check all food for mold and other signs of spoilage. If in doubt, throw it out. Use only bottled water for eating and drinking until local authorities verify that the public tap water system is safe to use again. You can purify water by boiling it vigorously—it should be bubbling and rolling for at least one minute. If you can't boil water, add six drops of ordinary, unscented household bleach per gallon of contaminated water and stir well. Let the water stand for thirty minutes before use. Bleach alone will not kill parasitic organisms or make the water potable.

CHAPTER TWO

WILDFIRES

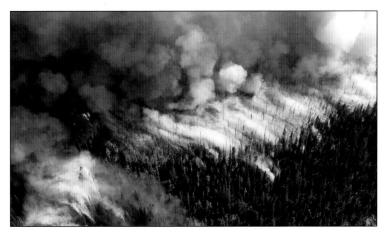

Widespread wildfire. *Credit: Pixabay.*

Each year, wildfires burn more than a million acres of forest and woodland. Wildfires usually start from lightning, cigarettes, matches, burning debris, sparks from a car or train exhaust, campfires, or arson. Unfortunately, most of the time—as much as 90 percent of the time according to the US Department of Interior—humans cause wildfires. You might think that wildfires only occur in dry, hot climates or deep in a forest but they can happen just about anywhere. We live in Amarillo/

Texas Panhandle and we have a "grassfire" season where huge swaths of land are constantly at risk because of fast-spreading wildfire.

Wildfires take place around the world and in most of the fifty states. These infernos are most common in the West, where heat, drought, and frequent and violent thunderstorms create ideal wildfire conditions. Some of the worst conflagrations take place in Montana, Idaho, Wyoming, Washington, Colorado, Oregon, and California. 2017 was likely the costliest for wildfires in US history because of dry conditions ripe for wildfires; it saw nearly 53,000 wildfires in the United States and over ten million acres went up in flames. Over 4.5 million US homes were identified at high or extreme risk of wildfire, with more than two million in California alone. At one time, there were an astonishing twenty-seven wildfires burning across the West. The December California wildfires were some of the worst in that state's history, fueled by dry conditions, serious Santa Ana winds, and plenty of wooded areas. If you watched videos of the fires, then you know how surreal the images seemed, how furious and destructive they were.

AccuWeather has predicted that the economic toll of the 2017 wildfire season in California alone would reach $180 billion (no exact amount is available at the time of this writing). Imagine what goes into that estimate: homes damaged or lost (and many of them were in expensive neighborhoods); business and school closures; clogged commuter routes; respiratory illnesses from the bad air; costs to fight the fires and rehabilitation costs; lost sales, business activity, and workdays lost. (Side note: Canada had its worst wildfire season in sixty years in 2017.)

Wildfires can travel at amazing speeds, up to 14 miles per hour with the right fuel and wind conditions. Don't think that because you aren't adjacent to a grass field or a forest that you are safe from a wildfire. Sparks and embers can travel a mile or more.

Three conditions need to be present in order for a wildfire to burn, a relationship known as the fire triangle: fuel, oxygen, and a heat source. Fuel is any flammable material surrounding a fire, including trees, grasses, brush, even homes. The greater an area's fuel load, the more intense the fire. Air supplies the oxygen a fire needs to burn.

Heat sources help spark the wildfire and bring fuel to temperatures hot enough to ignite. Lightning, burning campfires or cigarettes, hot winds, and even the sun can all provide sufficient heat to spark a wildfire. The weather conditions for a wildfire occur when dry weather and drought convert green vegetation into bone-dry, flammable fuel, strong winds spread fire quickly over land, and warm temperatures encourage combustion. When these factors come together, all that's needed is a spark — in the form of lightning, arson, a downed power line, or a burning campfire or cigarette.

Traditional methods for extinguishing existing wildfires include dousing it with water and spraying fire retardants. Firefighters fight these wildfires by depriving them of one or more of the fire triangle fundamentals. The fire triangle's three components are the three basic and necessary elements of fire: heat, fuel, and oxidization. Remove any of the three elements, and the fire is extinguished.

Firefighters frequently clear vegetation to create firebreaks (obstacles to the spread of fire) so the fire is deprived of fuel. Doing so often slows or contains the fire. Prescribed fires are another way to control wildfires. This is done by deliberately starting fires and the idea behind

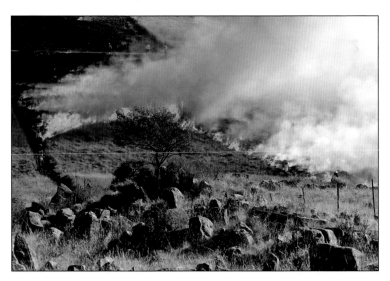

Firefighters monitor a prescribed burn. *Credit: Pixabay.*

controlled burning is to remove undergrowth, brush, and ground litter from a forest, in which case you deprive a wildfire of fuel.

Preparation

Your preparation should include 1) analysis of risk to your property and family; 2) proactive precautionary actions; and 3) family emergency management plan. Wildfires can move so quickly that the odds are that you may not be at your property when you are endangered. But let us look first at preparing your house or building.

Make sure your property adheres to all local fire codes, building codes, and weed abatement ordinances. Are there modifications you can make to your home now or in the future? Is your home built of flame-resistant materials? In high wildfire areas, more and more homes are being built or remodeled to reduce the fire risk. Your roof construction is the most important fire-resistant choice to make with your house, be it using metal, tile, or slate.

The Ready, Set, Go model (below) shows homeowners how to fire-proof their homes through several techniques:

- Use 1/8-inch screens to cover vents to prevent embers from entering attics or other part of the house.
- The next time you put on a new roof, use non-combustible materials such as metal, slate, or tile.
- Make sure your home has a one-hundred-foot defensible space cleared of brush and other dry vegetation that will go up in a fire.

For the exterior, think about using brick, stone, or concrete, since those materials each are more resistant to fire than wood. You can find commercial fire retardants for your wood exterior. To begin preparing, you should build an emergency kit and make a family communications plan.

What should your emergency plan consist of?

- Emergency supplies
- Defensible plan
- Family communication and alternate route options

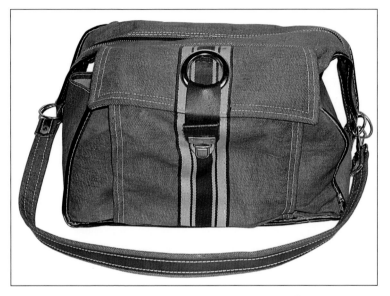

Pack an emergency travel bag, filled with supplies.

Emergency supplies

Don't wait until the last minute to prepare. Start right now. Find a back-pack or small carry bag to load up with all your supplies. Start with a complete first-aid kit, and possibly add burn cream and other ointments that might help someone who was injured by the fire. Make copies of your important documents, medications list, and personal identifica-tion for each family member. Assume that if you have to evacuate, you will be away from your home for an extended period of time. Each fam-ily member needs to have an accessible emergency supply kit/bag to take with them. Depending on how much lead time you have there are things that will not fit into your backpack (such as water jugs). Here's a list of components for your emergency supplies:

Emergency Supply Kit Checklist

- A sturdy pair of shoes and a flashlight in case of a sudden evacuation at night.
- A map of your surrounding area. This sounds antiquated but you need a map for your locality. Yes, a paper map. What if the power is out or cell-phone service interrupted? Get a map and mark at least two evacuation routes by car and two by foot.
- Extra eyeglasses or contact lenses.
- Copies of important documents (birth certificates, passports, etc.).
- A three-day supply of non-perishable food (jerky, powdered soups, backpack-style freeze-dried packages, protein and breakfast bars).
- Three gallons of water per person. If three gallons per person is too much for each backpack, at least put in two bottles of water each and have a couple of jugs of water in your trunk or near the door.
- Prescriptions or special medications.
- Change of clothing: underwear, T-shirt, socks, deodorant, shampoo or body wash, washrag, and small towel.
- An extra set of car keys, credit cards, and cash or traveler's checks.
- First-aid kit.
- Flashlight.
- Battery-powered radio and extra batteries. We suggest a hand-crank flashlight, and a hand-crank radio in case your batteries go bad.
- Sanitation supplies (hand wipes, toilet paper, hand sanitizer, etc.).
- Don't forget pet food and water!

Items to take if time allows:

- Easily carried valuables such as family photos, flash drives, and other irreplaceable but small items. If you go by car, take your laptop but if you're on foot, leave it.

- Chargers for your cell phones, laptops, etc.
- A small power unit for emergency charges for your phones.
- A second emergency backpack in your car in case you aren't home when a wildfire hits.

Emergency Action Plan

Study your map and find two reasonable, safe evacuation driving routes and two walking routes in case your car fails or the streets don't allow a car to proceed. It's likely that if you are evacuated, the emergency management teams will already have your route laid out but you need to be prepared just in case. Drive each route at least once with your family to familiarize them with it.

What if you were somehow injured and someone else had to drive you to safety? Determine a designated emergency meeting location for your family outside the fire area. A church, a mall, or somewhere notable are all ideal meeting places. This is how you can be certain that everyone is safely evacuated. Designate a friend or family member that is not in your area as a point of contact. They will act as a contact point and be a single source of communication in case your family is separated or your local communications are shut down or overloaded.

Don't forget your pets or livestock. If you can't move them in time, leave them means of escape or evacuation. Show all your family members how to shut off the gas, propane, and electricity in case you're not home when the wildfire approaches. Keep several fire extinguishers on hand in your house, train your family to use them, and check them regularly.

How can you protect your home or building while you're gone? Begin with creating defensible space. A defensible space is one of the most effective and certainly most cost-effective means to combat potential wildfires. A defensible space is an area around your home or building where combustible fuel is removed or ameliorated so that the closer you get to your house, the less there is to burn. Having a defensible space will also provide room to work for those fighting the fire.

First, how much defensible space do you have around your property right now? Is there considerable vegetation around your house? Are there things that could catch fire easily and put your house in danger? Think in terms of preventative anti-fire zones and in those zones, think about both horizontal and vertical protection. For example purposes, you have the three concentric zones of defensible space: Zones 1, 2, and 3.

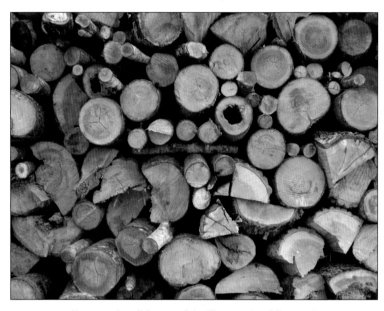

Keep combustible materials, like stacks of firewood, a safe distance from your home.

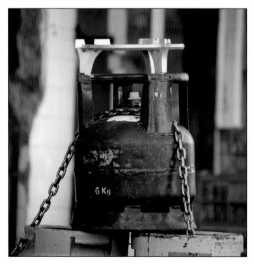

Move propane tanks to a safe location away from dwellings.
Credit: Pixabay.

Zone 1 is the area within thirty feet of your home or building. The idea is to eliminate fire-prone vegetation and remove all combustible materials. What constitutes combustible materials? A big stack of fire-wood for starters. Do you have lumber decking? A big propane tank? Piles of leaves? Open barrel-full of trash? Even things like your patio furniture, umbrella, leftover lumber from that big project you never finished. Anything that can burn and put your house or building in danger is a combustible material. Get rid of it or modify it.

Quick notes on things you can do to improve your defensible space:

- Trim trees and shrub limbs so they do not come into contact with electrical wires. Don't let limbs hang over your chimney.
- Be careful around power lines. Hire a professional to trim around power lines so you don't make a mistake with your life.
- Clean your gutters, chimneys, and your roof from pine needles, leaves, and other flammable material.
- Store flammable or combustible material in approved containers.
- Prune all lower branches 8 feet from the ground.
- Check all your trees in Zone 1 for dead or dying branches and remove them.
- If firefighters have to come into your neighborhood, they will need to see the house numbers, so keep them clear and viewable from the street.

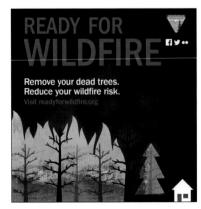

A reminder on the Bureau of Land Management's website to remove dead trees well before wildlife season. *Credit: The Bureau of Land Management.*

Zone 1

Build in natural firebreaks, areas where there are no vegetation or burnable elements. Assess both the horizontal and vertical aspects of vegetation when designing your defensible space. Wildland vegetation such as grass, brush, and timber is extremely combustible. Even landscape vegetation is a hazard. Vegetation is your biggest burn threat in Zone 1.

Thin out those canopied trees near your house, meaning any trees within fifty to seventy-five feet near the house. Prune branches up to ten-feet high and eliminate all shrubs at the base of the trunks. Remove any accumulation of dead leaves. Fires can move horizontally from bush to bush and tree to tree but also vertically where the fire spreads to the tops of trees and creates what is known as a crown fire.

Zone 2

This second zone has more clumps of trees and shrubs than Zone 1 but not as much as Zone 3. Limit this zone to a few islands of vegetation but again, limit combustible plants or buildings or fuel.

Driveways and paved or gravel walkways and patios are hard break options that create firebreaks throughout your yard in Zone 2. Plant fire-resistant, low-volume vegetation. Prune dead branches. Outside buildings such as a detached garage, pump house, pergola, or a tool shed should be at least forty to sixty feet from your house, more if it holds combustible materials. If you are building it new, it's easy to comply with recommended construction practices that increase fire resistance. Place wood piles at least thirty feet from the building and store the wood in a vegetation-free zone such as a graveled area.

Zone 3

Reduce any fuels that are farther than one hundred feet from your house by thinning and pruning vegetation horizontally and vertically. Your goals in Zone 3 are to help slow an approaching wildfire. Zone 3 should also be an aesthetic transition between the more heavily modified Zone 2 and the unmodified surroundings beyond Zone 3.

So you have taken all the more permanent precautions but you've found out a fire is coming your way. You have some lead time. What now? If time permits, there are a number of things you can do to keep the building as safe as possible.

- Shut off any and all fuel lines, including propane, natural gas, and oil.
- Move curtains and fabric-covered furniture away from windows and sliding doors. If the glass breaks, you do not want anything flammable near the window/door.
- Remove any combustible objects from the yard, especially gas grills and fuel cans, and discard them as far from your structure and any nearby structures as possible. You should also move any stacks of firewood as far from the building as possible.
- If time permits, trim grass and vegetation as low to the ground as possible around the building and any external propane tanks. This will help reduce the combustible material that would allow the fire to reach you or the fuel source.

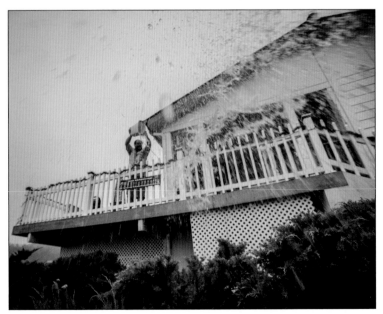

A man saturates his home and vegetation with water in hopes of keeping sparks at bay. *Credit: Lance Cheung, USDA.*

Try to wet the area. If the building has hoses and running water, utilize that water to create a safer structure. Remember that water may not necessarily stop a fire, but it will slow it down.

- Use hoses or sprinklers to saturate the roof of the building, the walls, and the ground immediately surrounding the building.
- Fill any large containers present with water (if possible), and surround the perimeter of the building with them.

<u>What can you do to avoid starting a wildfire?</u>

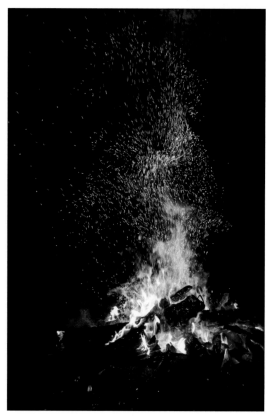

Never leave a campfire unattended.

- Never leave a campfire unattended. Completely extinguish the fire—by dousing it with water and stirring the ashes until cold—before sleeping or leaving the campsite.

- Follow local ordinances when burning yard waste. Avoid backyard burning in windy conditions, and keep a shovel nearby, have access to water, or fire retardant nearby.

- If you spot a wildfire, call 911, your local fire department, or the park service immediately. Try to note the location and, if possible, take a quick snapshot of the fire and a screenshot of the GPS.

- Never leave a fire unattended—not a campfire, not a debris fire, and not a barrel fire. Make sure you completely extinguish the fire and the only real way to do it right is to use a lot of water.

- Be careful when camping when fueling your stoves, lanterns, and heaters. Don't re-fuel your device if it is hot. Don't spill flammable liquids anywhere near the devices or anything else that is combustible.

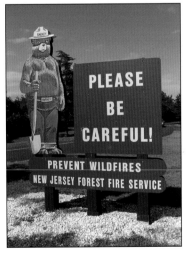

- Cigarettes, cigars, and other things you might be smoking—don't toss them while driving. Don't toss them in grass as you walk along the road. If you are in a national or state park, in the forest, be extra careful and don't extinguish it with cavalier flair. Completely extinguish your smoke before discarding it.

- If you are burning trash, follow local ordinances. Be careful. Be observant. Don't burn in windy

Smokey Bear reminds campers in New Jersey to use caution. *Credit: Pixabay.*

conditions. Keep a shovel nearby and have a water source and/or fire retardant handy.

Survival

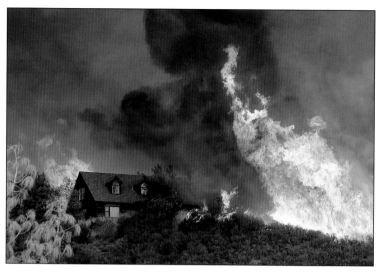

Mountainside home in the path of a devastating California wildfire.

Evacuation is vital to survival. If you aren't there, you only lose your property, not your life. So get out early. But if you don't leave, the experts say, it's actually better to stay than to run at the last minute. Nationally, emergency declarations by government to evacuate, even if mandatory, are not always enforceable. Don't be one of the citizens they have to convince to leave. Staying puts firefighters and first responders at risk if they have to come rescue you.

Get to know your local and national weather and emergency alerts. This is your lifeline to staying safe. The National Weather Service provides active alerts on weather across the nation. NOAA Weather Radio provides 24/7 information on watches, warnings, and advisories from the National Weather Service.

The Emergency Alert System broadcasts flash flood warnings on commercial radio and TV. Wireless Emergency Alerts (WEA) are emergency messages sent by authorized government alerting authorities through your mobile carrier, and they include flash flood warnings. FEMA has also launched an app that provides email alerts and text messages to the general public. Third party sources that deliver email and weather alerts are plentiful and pop up every day or so it seems.

We discovered two slightly controversial wildfire-survival shelters:

1. Emergency wildfire bags you carry with you and use only as a last resort. These emergency shelters look like aluminized sleeping bags and are designed to withstand temperatures of 500 degrees Fahrenheit (260 degrees Celsius). These fire blankets are supposed to provide a high degree of protection against radiant heat but if the fire comes in direct contact with the aluminum covering, then that shelter will not protect you at all.
2. Fire bunkers or fire pods. Experts are skeptical of these because they are not regulated, generally untested and depends on if the bunker is above or below ground. Some companies will build these into your house construction which is good because if you have to leave your house to get in one, you put yourself and others in danger.

Both of these seem promising but need more evidence of success.

If you have to evacuate

If you get the message to evacuate, don't hesitate. Time is of the essence. Quickly shut off all gas appliances as well as the main gas valve, and electrical to your home. Prop a ladder against your house so if the firefighters need to get on your roof to put out a fire. Have hoses attached, and if you have time, fill up some buckets of water.

Grab your family, your wildfire action bags, and your pets, and get out. Know your evacuation route. You've planned for this after all. Don't panic. Be purposeful and efficient. When the fire is closing in and pressure is mounting, you may forget to grab your supply backpack and where to go. Put a cap and jacket on and wear closed shoes to protect from flying fire, sparks, ashes, etc.

As you drive, if the fire is within view, keep your windows up to avoid embers and smoke and recycle air conditioning. The ashes and smoke create wind currents that move low to the ground, which means an active wildfire can transmit burning embers up to a mile ahead of the actual fire. So keep your eyes alert for any new fires or for new directions of the existing fire. Turn the radio to local stations or emergency stations to get the latest information. Drive with your headlights and hazard lights on so other evacuees can see you through any smoke. Passengers should be vigilant for pedestrians, livestock, fleeing animals, and stalled cars. There could be lots of smoke so all need to share in prevention. Be sure to follow directions of law enforcement at all times.

If you did not get the order to evacuate

The wildfire you've been preparing for (and dreading) is here. You are in your house. You should have already done this, but if not, go turn off the gas supply to reduce the chances of explosion.

Keep tuned to the television and to the radio for the latest emergency information. If you have a short-wave radio, you can find the channel for emergency personnel to keep up with firefighters, police, and other local emergency management.

Secure your pets inside. Turn off the air conditioning or air circulation system. Detach electrical garage doors. Back your car into the garage and leave the keys in the ignition—you don't want to be looking for your car keys if you need to make a quick getaway.

Close your windows so you don't get a draft and bring the fire into the house. Move upholstered furniture and any other flammables away from windows and doors. In case smoke gets in your house, turn on all your lights and put flashlights in each room. If the fire is close, take down flammable drapes and curtains. Be ready to evacuate all family members and pets if the evacuation request comes in.

Listen and watch for air quality reports and health warnings about smoke. Close all windows and doors to prevent outside smoke from getting in. If you have asthma or another lung disease, follow your health-care provider's advice and seek medical care if your symptoms worsen.

You still might have to evacuate of your own volition so assess each of the evacuation options to find your safest and most advantageous escape route, and decide under what circumstances you will choose to evacuate. Will you drive or walk? Most every time the answer will be drive but there are situations where walking may be quicker and/or safer. The most dangerous places to be are uphill from the flames, downwind from the fire; this essentially means stay upwind of the fire.

If you leave by car, don't cut it too close. Many injuries and deaths occur when people wait too long to leave and cut it close, leaving a small margin for error. You might drive off the road, into a tree, into a lake,

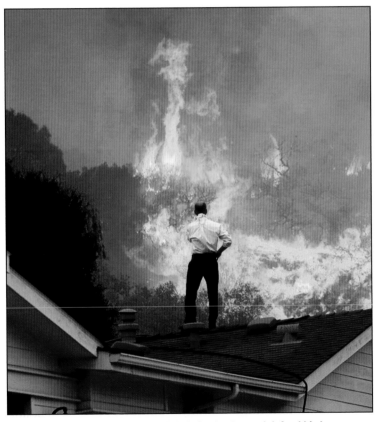

A man makes the controversial choice to stay and defend his home during a wildfire. *Credit: Jeff Hill.*

have a falling tree land on you, or hit a power line. So if you leave by car, do so in plenty of time.

There is a small controversial movement, that maintains that if you have prepared an effective defensible space (Zones 1, 2, and 3) and if you have proper water supply and the courage to fight fire, you should stay and defend your property. The idea is that those pesky small fires that hit a roof or a small bush or debris pile, if unattended, can grow into a much bigger fire and destroy your house. If you are there, they contend, you could easily put those fires out and keep your homestead safe. The problem is, the second leading cause of death in woodland fires is people staying outside to defend their homes. Unless you have firefighting experience, and unless you have firefighting suits and equipment, this strategy is not for you. Leave early and hope your defensible space is as efficient as you designed.

Let's say you miss the window of escape and the wildfire is near. Stay in your house.

If you are trapped in your house or building

If you become trapped in the house or perhaps you are forced to take shelter in a building, stay inside no matter what. If the fire surrounds the building, you're more likely to survive inside than outside. The killer in wildfires is radiant heat.

Stay calm. Getting agitated or excited will impede your leadership, constrict your decision-making abilities, and generally interfere with your ability to survive. If you have time, change your clothes from nylon (jogging suits and hosiery, especially) to cotton. Nylon has a low melting point. It'll melt to your skin in the heat.

Close doors, windows, vents, and any other openings so you don't get a draft that will spread the fire to the inside. Don't lock the doors, because you may need to get out or firefighters may need to get in. Get to an interior room and stay away from exterior walls. If you are with others, stick together, don't separate.

If you are trapped outside of your house, out in the open

If you can't outrun it or if you're surrounded, the safest thing to do is quickly locate a building or vehicle, or a body of water (a pool, a lake or pond, a river). Get in. Swim across the river if you can. Wet your clothing if there is water. Every second counts so keep your head about you and be efficient in action. Use a road as a barrier if possible; this will buy you time.

If you locate a building or vehicle, look for anything to cover your body—a heavy canvas tarp (not plastic or nylon) or a blanket. Again, wet it down if possible. If you find mud or wet soil, use that to cover exposed parts of your body, especially your neck, head and face. And use a shirt or other material as a filter to breathe through. Wet the cloth if you can.

Remember that wildfires can travel up to 14 miles per hour. You can't run that fast. If it's close, get face down in a ditch or a low-lying area. Protect your airways. This is the most important thing you can do. Even if the fire passes over you, you still have a chance of escaping if you can breathe. Once you inhale smoke and carbon monoxide, you risk passing out and dying.

If you are trapped in your car:

If you have no choice but to remain with your car during a fire front but cannot drive because there is no route, do the following in order to survive:

- Roll up all of the car windows and close all the air vents.
- Put the air conditioning on re-circulation.
- Leave the engine running even when you stop.
- Don't worry about the gas tank. Vehicles with metal gas tank rarely explode. You are much safer staying inside the car than you would be on foot if the fire is that bad.
- Keep the radio on so that you know what direction the fire is heading and where it is focused. Use a compass and other navigation aids so that you can get out of the fire as quickly as possible.

When you stop driving, park behind a solid structure if possible. This will help to block radiant heat, which is deadly. If you cannot find a solid structure to take the heat, then stop your car in a clear area beside the road or in a similar suitable place.

So after all this research about being trapped in your car by wildfire, the most common expertise offered is this: your car will not protect you and, in fact, will boil you alive. If a wildfire is all around you, the heat and smoke unbearable, it would be hard to imagine purposefully exiting the vehicle to face the elements, naked, so to speak.

You see a vehicle that is not your vehicle, and the fire is approaching quickly. When your choices are running on foot or using a vehicle, opt for the vehicle. Yes, you are taking someone else's car to save your life. It's still extremely dangerous, but will give you better odds of surviving than being on foot. Look, if the fire consumes the car, you're not going to make it. Cars are not great shelters against fires. And don't steal a car unless it's clear that it's abandoned and no one else needs it to escape.

But be careful. A car will heat up and boil you alive if you are in it. Think of how hot metal gets. You must avoid being caught in a vehicle because a car offers no protection from radiant heat. Think of how fast a covered pot of water reaches a boil, and you have a good idea of why cars are not a safe place to be during a fire.

Once the fire has passed, it is time to get out of the car.

- Immediately attend to children and anyone experiencing stress or shock.
- If you have a cell phone and service, call for help immediately.
- If the car is still operational then drive away from the fire to safety. If the car is no longer operational walk away from the fire to seek help.

How to Survive a Wildfire on Foot

The most dangerous places to be in relation to a wildfire are uphill from the flames and downwind from the fire. Always try to stay upwind of the fire. So if the wind is blowing past you and toward the fire, run into the wind. If the wind is behind the fire and blowing toward you, run perpendicular to the fire so that you are escaping both the flames and the course those flames will blow towards. Head for non-flammable terrain (parking lot, stadium, wide road, etc.) If at all possible, head for the nearest, biggest area that is unlikely to burn. While the fire might be wide, it still needs combustible material like trees, brush, and tall grass to burn.

- Look for areas free of trees and brush. Always try to put a body of water between you and the fire.
- Places which have already burned are sometimes the safest places to go. That said, make sure that the area is completely extinguished before proceeding.
- Avoid high-burn places such as fields of dry grass, forests, canyons, barren plowed fields, riverbeds, ponds, and rocky areas. And as the fire advances, even if you've temporarily escaped, avoid places that could leave you trapped once the fire advances.
- Avoid places where you could get trapped by fire—ridges, canyons, ski slopes, and other elevated spots with no escape.
- If you are hiking in backcountry, look for a depression with sparse fuel. Lie face down in the depression. Stay down until after the fire passes.
- Choose downhill routes if possible. Fire moves faster uphill due to updrafts.
- A drainage pipe or an underground hole could be the place that saves your life. Lay low and curled up. Cover any exposed skin. This will also help reduce smoke inhalation.
- Seek emergency help as soon as possible. You might have thermal burns that need to be treated.

You need to breathe, so get low. In order to breathe the best air, stay as low to the ground as possible. Cover your nose and mouth with a wet cloth of some sort, and if not wet, a shirt or bandana or cloth, and hold it there until you get to a safer area.

If all else fails and you have to stand your ground, cover your body with anything that will protect you from the fire. Wet clothing, a wet blanket, anything except nylon or rubber. If you don't have anything else, cover yourself with dirt or mud. Get down and stay down. As hard as it sounds, stay covered until the fire passes. Failure to do this could get you killed.

If you are driving and you aren't yet trapped: If the vehicle can run and you're capable of driving it, then do so. Drive safely and slowly so you can clearly your surroundings and so that anyone else on the road can see you.

- Drive slowly.
- Turn your headlights on.
- Keep an eye peeled for other vehicles and pedestrians. Stop to let any endangered pedestrians you see ride along with you.
- Don't drive through heavy smoke.
- Don't stop until you are well clear of any danger but if you have to stop, do so in an inflammable area, such as a parking lot.

Aftermath

Exercise caution even after the fire. Don't return home until you're told it's safe to do so. When you get home, use caution. Is there any standing water outside? Are there any hotspots in your yard, any embers or smoldering debris on your roof? Stumps can burn for days or longer. The wind could come along and make the hotspot flare up.

Do you smell gas? Do you see any fallen power lines? If you judge it safe to go in, check the house before you just go turn on the gas, electrical, and water. If you see damage to any of those, consult a professional immediately. Check your attic for any hidden fire problems—embers or sparks—that could have burrowed through your roof. Continue to check regularly throughout your return for several days.

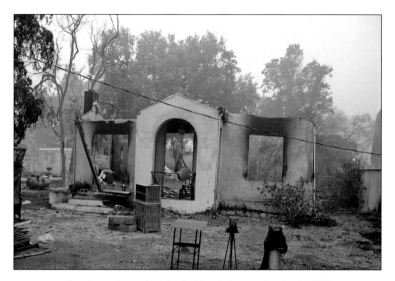

The charred remains of a California home. *Credit: Jeff Hill.*

Coming home after a wildfire can be difficult. It may have been weeks since you've been allowed back. Your home may be burned up beyond recognition. You may have neighbors who have lost their properties or lives. Everything you have worked for may be gone. Check with officials before attempting to return to your home. You don't want to risk going back in when there is still danger.

- Check grounds for hot spots, smoldering stumps, and vegetation that might still be vulnerable to sparks.
- Check your roof and all exterior areas for sparks or embers. Remove any loose limbs, leaves, or anything else that could catch fire from an errant ember.
- Check the attic and all through your house for any hidden burning sparks or embers.
- Open cabinets and smell vents. Be a detective. You don't want to lay your head on your pillow tonight if your house is a possible fire hazard.
- Turn off all appliances and make sure the meter is not damaged before turning on the main circuit breaker.

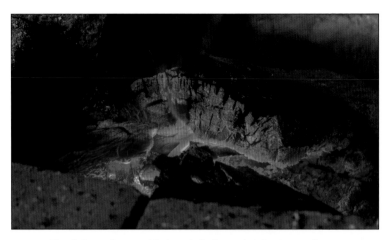

Check for embers and hot spots before returning to your home.

- If you sense fire danger, contact 911. Your neighborhood will thank you.
- Flash floods are a deadly hazard after a wildfire, because rain falling in a burned area upstream of your location has no vegetation or grass to stop it from heading down-hill. Stay away from ditches, streams, storm channels, and arroyos.
- Keep a battery-powered radio to listen for emergency updates, reports of weather and flash flooding, and news reports.
- You already have an evacuation plan in place, so if something goes wrong and winds cause fires again, make sure all family members know it in case you need to leave your home for any reason.
- Do not drink or use water from your faucet (or even your fridge water dispenser) until emergency officials give the thumbs up. Your water supply systems can be damaged during wildfires or flooding.
- As you move around your yard and drive in your burned neighborhood, be aware of and use extreme caution around

trees, power poles, and other tall objects that may have lost stability during the fire.

- Many burned structures and surfaces will be unstable. If the winds are up, be especially wary of trees, especially clearly-burned trees.

- If you try and you have no power, make sure the main breaker is on. If the breakers are on and power is still not turned on, contact the utility company.

- If you have a propane tank or system, contact a propane supplier, turn off valves on the system, and leave valves closed until the supplier inspects your system. If you have a heating oil tank system, contact a heating oil supplier for an inspection of your system before using.

- Before you start cleanup, document all damage with photographs. Contact your insurance agent and find out what to do next.

- For the next week, have all family members maintain a fire watch—and by that we mean smell and look for smoke or sparks throughout the house and on the rooftop, in gutters, in the yard, in the attic.

CHAPTER THREE

TORNADOES

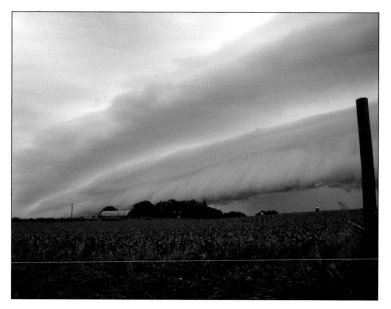

Storm cloud, Winnebago, Illinois. *Credit: NOAA, Janice Thompson*

Tornadoes are one of nature's most powerful forces, awesome and destructive, unpredictable and furious. Every state in America has at least one documented tornado. The United States sees an average of one thousand tornadoes in a year. Most tornadoes hit between 4 p.m. and 9 p.m.

in the evening in the warmer months but even so, tornadoes can occur at any time of day, and on any day of the year.

Tornadoes can be terrifying and capricious, destroying a row of homes but leaving one in the middle unscathed. Winds from tornadoes can reach speeds up to 250 to 280 miles per hour (the fastest wind speed recorded in a tornado is 302 miles per hour on May 3, 1999, near Bridge Creek, Oklahoma) and no doubt, you've seen evidence of what unimaginable damage they can do. You might have also seen odd and bizarre results from twisters like asphalt pavement stripped, wood splinters embedded into bricks, straw driven into trees.

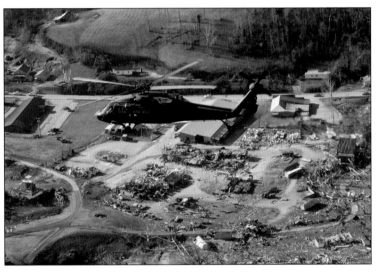

Helicopter view of tornado destruction over West Liberty, Kentucky.

So what is a tornado? According to the *Glossary of Meteorology* (AMS 2000), a tornado is "a violently rotating column of air, pendant from a cumuliform cloud or underneath a cumuliform cloud, and often (but not always) visible as a funnel cloud." For a vortex to be classified as a tornado, it must be in contact with the ground **and** the cloud base. When you see a rotation descend from a cloud, if it doesn't touch the ground, it is not officially a tornado.

So essentially, a tornado is a dark funnel-shaped cloud composed of violently-rotating winds. Tornadoes produce wind speeds of up to 300 miles per hour. The diameter of a tornado can vary between a few feet and a mile, and a tornado's track can extend from less than a mile to several hundred miles. Tornadoes generally travel in a northeast direction (depending on the prevailing winds) at speeds ranging from 20 to 60 miles per hour.

Meteorologists disagree about how to define and classify tornadoes. For example, the difference between a strong mesocyclone (parent thunderstorm circulation) on the ground, and a large, weak tornado is unclear. Scientists also have differing ideas on whether separate touchdowns of the same funnel constitute separate tornadoes. Is it possible

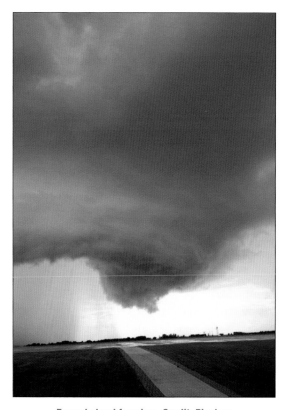

Funnel cloud forming. *Credit: Pixabay.*

for a tornado to not have a visible funnel? What wind speed of the cloud-to-ground vortex determines the genesis of a tornado? How close must two or more different tornadic circulations become to qualify as a one multiple-vortex tornado instead of separate tornadoes? There are no firm answers.

So how do tornadoes form? It's complicated. The classic answer is that tornadoes form when warm moist Gulf air meets dry air from the Rockies and cold Canadian air. Many thunderstorms do form under those conditions (near warm fronts, cold fronts, and drylines), but do not come close to producing tornadoes. Even when the large-scale environment is extremely favorable for tornadic thunderstorms, not every thunderstorm spawns a tornado. The most lethal and destructive tornadoes occur from supercells, rotating thunderstorms with a well-defined radar circulation called a mesocyclone. Supercells can also produce damaging hail, severe non-tornadic winds, unusually frequent lightning and flash floods. Mesocyclones dictate tornado formation. Tornado prediction is based on understanding the essential elements that come into play in order to forecast the storms that can produce tornadoes.

Some necessary ingredients for tornado formation:

1. A strong jet stream, as this provides the necessary vertical wind shear. Wind shear, an increase of wind speed with height, starts the funnel rotating.
2. A substantial amount of water vapor especially in the lower troposphere. When the moisture condenses in the lower troposphere, it releases most of the energy that drives the storm.
3. Lastly, you need warm, dry air in the middle altitudes. In Tornado Alley (roughly, the center of America, between the Rockies and Appalachians), air comes off the Mexican Plateau and caps a lid on the moist, warm air building in the lower atmosphere. In the Southern plains, solar energy almost literally cooks the water vapor but the cap prevents gradual release of this energy. Suddenly, an explosive

thunderstorm occurs out of the blue sky and starts to release this energy. This is the source of power for the convective storms that create thunder, lightning, and tornadoes.

FACTS

- The most powerful tornadoes occur in the United States.
- The typical tornado is fleeting, and will only last for a few minutes.
- Every tornado is unique and has its own color, sound, and shape.
- Average number of tornadoes per year in the United States (1950–2010): about 1,000.
- Five states with highest incidence of tornadoes (average per year, 1950–2007): Texas (139), Oklahoma (57), Kansas (55), Florida (55), Nebraska (45).
- States with lowest incidence of tornadoes (total number, 1950–2004): Alaska (2), Rhode Island (9), Hawaii (31), Vermont (37), Oregon (87).
- Most tornadoes in one month: 543 (May 2003).
- Most tornado deaths in one year: 519 (1953).
- Fewest tornado deaths in one year: 15 (1986).
- The chances that a tornado is a F5, the highest classification of destruction and power for a tornado on the F-scale, is less than 0.1 percent.
- Tornadoes can happen at any time of year, but they spawn most during the spring and early summer. In numbers of tornadoes, the peak months are May and June. April is the deadliest month.
- May holds the record for experiencing the most tornadoes. In May 2003, there were an unbelievable 543 recorded tornadoes.

- On average, sixty people die each year as a result of tornadoes. The mythology from movies is that deaths in tornadoes occur from getting sucked up and spun out of control but in fact, most deaths happen due to collapsing buildings, car accidents, and flying and falling debris.
- A tornado watch means weather conditions are prime for a tornado.
- A tornado warning means a tornado has been sighted or indicated by radar.
- Tornadoes are caused by cold air blowing over an area of warm air, causing it to violently rise.
- Tornadoes most frequently occur in the late afternoon and evening.
- Oklahoma City has been hit by more tornadoes than any other place.
- Early season tornadoes tend to be more intense, on average, than those that occur later.
- Early season tornadoes most often occur after dark because the daylight hours are shorter. Since tornadoes are more difficult to identify at night, more people are caught unaware in early season.
- Don't let the movie *Twister* inform your knowledge of how tornadoes act. That's the movies! Oh, and do not tie yourself to a pole to survive a tornado like Bill Paxton and Helen Hunt. Dumb move.
- Tornado Alley describes an area in the middle of the United States that is prone to tornadoes. The region is loosely between the Rocky Mountains and Appalachian Mountains. This is not an official weather term but one popularized by the media.
- Which states have the most tornadoes? According to the National Climatic Data Center, Texas reports the

highest number of tornadoes. Kansas (think Dorothy and Toto) and Oklahoma are second and third, respectively.

- Around the world, latitudes between about 30 degrees and 50 degrees North or South provide the most favorable environment for tornadoes.
- The direction in which a tornado twists depends a lot upon which hemisphere you're in. Generally, most tornadoes in the northern hemisphere rotate cyclonically, or counter-clockwise. Only around five percent of tornadoes in the northern hemisphere rotate clockwise, or anti-cyclonically. In the southern hemisphere, however, most tornadoes rotate clockwise.

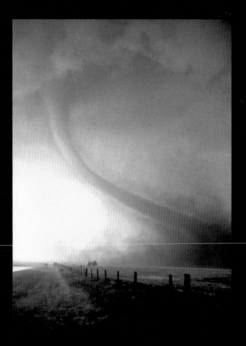

Oklahoma tornado illuminated by the sun. *Credit: NOAA.*

Ten deadliest tornadoes

Date	Intensity	States affected	Deaths
March 18, 1925	F5	MO, IL, IN	695
May 6, 1840	Unknown	LA, MS	317
May 27, 1896	F4	MO, IL	255
April 5, 1936	F5	MS	216
April 6, 1936	F4	GA	203
April 9, 1947	F5	TX, KS, OK	181
May 22, 2011	EF5	MO	158
April 24, 1908	F4	LA, MS	143
June 12, 1899	F5	WI	117
June 8, 1953	F5	MI	116

Source: National Climatic Data Center.

You've seen the ratings tornadoes are given by scientists and perhaps you've been confused. You are not alone. The Fujita scale classifies tornadoes according to the damage they cause, not the size or wind speed (although this is most often correlative to damage). Almost half of all tornadoes fall into the F1 or "moderate damage" category. These tornadoes reach speeds of 73 to 112 miles per hour and can overturn automobiles and mobile homes, rip off the roofs of houses, and uproot trees. Only about 1 percent of tornadoes are classified as F5, meaning that they cause *incredible damage*. With wind speeds in excess of 261 miles per hour, these tornadoes are capable of lifting houses off their foundations and hurling them considerable distances. The scale goes as high as F12, theoretically, but since an F5 does as much damage as is possible, it's unlikely you'll ever see one rated any higher.

If you've ever seen a tornado forming or one in full form, then you know it's a frightening sight. But how do you know that what is unfolding in front of you is indeed a tornado and not just severe weather? Predicting tornadoes is difficult. Nationally, every single day, meteorologists at the NOAA Storm Prediction Center (SPC) issue daily forecasts for organized severe thunderstorms all over the United States based on current weather observations and forecast models. They also closely monitor areas they think are at a higher risk for tornadoes. If conditions develop that are favorable for tornadoes, SPC forecasters issue a severe thunderstorm or tornado watch. These watches typically last four to six hours. Local forecast offices, emergency managers, storm spotters, and the public are alerted to the possibility of severe weather. Tornado warnings are issued by the local National Weather Service Forecast Office when a tornado has been sighted or indicated by weather radar.

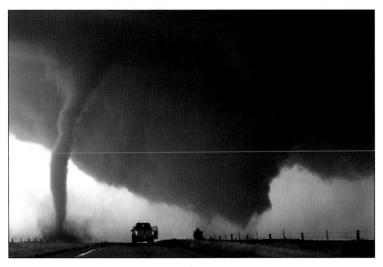

Storm spotting.
Credit: 2015 NOAA Weather in Focus Photo Contest, Brent Koops.

For starters, be alert during tornado season. Listen to or watch the weather (or easier, check any number of weather apps on your phone or tablet). Let's say you missed seeing the news or looking at your apps. Here are some hints that a tornado may be brewing and ready to touch down. Not all of these may happen but together, they are indicators:

- Strong rotation visible in the cloud base.
- Greenish, dark sky. When you see this, you'll see a color green you've never seen before. Almost anyone who has seen this sky describes it as eerie.
- Large high wall of clouds.
- Hail (and often large hail).
- A visible funnel-shaped cloud.
- A loud roaring sound (some say like a train), sustained cacophony, stronger than just consistent high wind.
- A sudden stillness or very calm wind during an ongoing storm.
- Small, bright flashes at ground level under a thunderstorm in the distance could be a tornado snapping power lines.
- Strong, persistent rotation in the cloud base.
- Whirling dust or debris on the ground under a cloud base—tornadoes sometimes have no funnel.
- Hail or heavy rain followed by either dead calm or a fast, intense wind shift. Many tornadoes are cloaked in heavy precipitation and can't be seen.
- At night, you'll see the cloud base, illuminated or silhouetted by lightning lowering over and over. The illumination can be lightning or if it's blue-green, it's likely from power lines being snapped from high winds.

Preparation

Many people are deathly afraid of tornadoes and rightfully so. But what are your odds of being struck by a tornado or worse, being killed by one? According to www.bookofodds.com, the chances of being killed by a tornado are one in 4,513,000. For comparison, the chances of dying from falling off a cliff: one in 4,101,000. By the same token, the odds of getting struck by lightning are one in 835,500.

Even if you lived in the same place in America for a long time, say in Tornado Alley, statistically, you'd have to wait nearly fifteen hundred years before being struck by a tornado. The "point probability" of direct strike by a tornado is small. But there are an awful lot of tornadoes and "points" in the United States, so during the peak of the season at least five tornadoes a day touch down somewhere in America.

You need a plan. You need a plan to survive tornados whether you live in Tornado Alley or any other part of North America. People who live in places where tornadoes rarely occur don't always see the need for a tornado plan. But tornadoes happen in every state at some point.

At home, you will want to have a family tornado plan in place. This sounds corny but if you want to survive, everything counts: Practice a family tornado drill at least once a year. Flying debris is the greatest danger in tornadoes, so store protective coverings (e.g., mattress, sleeping bags, thick blankets, etc.) in or next to your shelter space, ready to use on a moment's notice. Know where you can take shelter in a matter of seconds.

Buy yourself a National Oceanic and Atmospheric Administration (NOAA) Weather Radio. While the local media (radio or television) are a great source of relaying National Weather Service (NWS) tornado watches and warnings, they are only useful if you happen to have them turned on. The NOAA weather radio is on standby all the time, and will sound an alarm the moment a tornado watch or warning has been issued. If you are expecting severe weather, turn up the volume so you can clearly hear the alert (especially important if you are a sound sleeper).

Honestly, the best form of alert is you. Be cognizant of the surrounding conditions. Watch or check the weather every so often every day to anticipate the likelihood of severe weather. Make it an integrated part of your life to know what's going on. Be vigilant, especially in the spring when tornadoes most frequently occur.

If your home does not have a safe place that can be used as a tornado shelter (for instance, mobile homes), find out where the recommended shelter is in your neighborhood. Most mobile home parks, neighborhoods, and subdivisions should have a severe weather plan in place. Point of emphasis: mobile homes and tornadoes do not get along. They are not worthy structures against the power and fury of a tornado. If you have time, get out and away from your trailer.

So-called "safe rooms" are reinforced small rooms usually built in the interior of a home, (but more and more common in buildings) which are fortified by concrete and/or steel to offer extra protection against tornadoes, hurricanes, and other severe windstorms. These are common in areas frequented by tornadoes and they can be built in a basement. If no basement is available, on the ground floor. In existing homes, interior bathrooms or closets can be fortified into "safe rooms" as well.

Twister-pods and other kinds of survival pods are another option. They aren't cheap and it's almost the same cost prohibitively to build as an underground shelter. But if you don't have the inclination to build an underground shelter, the pod design may be for you.

At work, ask your employer for a copy of their severe weather safety plan. They should have a location where employees can seek shelter in the event of a tornado or other severe weather. If they don't have one or the other, get a team together, make it a priority, and create one. Don't let your safety rely on someone else's lack of preparation.

Tornado Survival Kit

You need to have at least one tornado kit per household. We carry one in each vehicle and have one at the house. We are lucky to have employers who take tornadoes seriously and we have plans, safe rooms, and tornado kits. Not all tornado kits are created equal but at the least, your kit should include:

- A battery-powered radio (preferably with weather channels).
- A flashlight in working order (do not store with batteries installed); there are battery-free flashlights now available.
- Immediate first-aid needs (bandages, antibiotic wipes, tweezers, etc.).

- Food (energy bars for certain) and a few bottles of water—make sure it's packaged, non-perishable food, but consider rotating provisions out every now and again to keep them fresh.
- Small, packaged, emergency thermal blankets.
- Cash and change (the ATMs may be out of cash in an emergency, or the power could be out).
- Large marking pen or bottle of spray paint (to write your address on the driveway or remains of structures for rescue personnel). In more gruesome situations, you may need to mark bodies or your own body with pertinent information.
- Copies of any critical medical records for you and for your family.
- Any medicines you take daily or frequently.
- Whistle (to help rescuers locate you).
- Place your tornado kit inside the place you have designated as your tornado shelter.
- Write down all important phone numbers, addresses, and other information you keep in your phone. Your phone could die, get wet, destroyed, or lost and where would you be without it? Do you remember phone numbers anymore? Nobody does, so keep a written record. And take a pic of the numbers to put them each in your phone contacts.
- If you own a home with a concrete foundation, a water/fire-proof safe that you bolt to the house foundation for storage of any irreplaceable documents is a good choice. These documents should be in the safe at all times. Do not wait until a tornado warning is issued before trying to put things in the safe.

I know we all live busy lives and for a family to stop and get together just to practice a tornado drill is asking a lot, but it's worth it. Imagine the flood after Hurricane Harvey and how many families wish they had practiced and talked about plans. Weather emergencies occur all over the country, all year long, and it just makes sense to have everyone on the same page, the same plan.

At least once per year for your family, school, or workplace, take the time to sit down and talk about what the plan is if a tornado warning confronts you. Ensure that everyone knows what to do without having to think about it.

All administrators of schools, shopping centers, nursing homes, hospitals, sports arenas, and other locations should regularly run well-coordinated drills. If you are planning to build a house, consider an underground tornado shelter or an interior safe room. This will be covered further in the Aftermath section, but any plans need to include a pre-determined place to meet after a disaster, as well as contact information and instructions.

Tornado Watch

A tornado watch defines an area where tornadoes and other kinds of severe weather are possible in the next several hours. Watch for a parallelogram logo when the meteorologist explains the power of the storm during a newscast. A watch does not mean tornadoes are imminent, just that you need to be alert, and to be prepared to go to safe shelter if tornadoes do happen or a warning is issued. This is the time to turn on local TV or radio, check your local weather apps, turn on and set the alarm switch on your weather radio, make sure you have ready access to safe shelter, be ready to implement your family tornado plan and make your friends and family aware of the potential for tornadoes in the area.

When a watch is issued: A watch is issued when atmospheric conditions are favorable for the formation of tornado producing thunderstorms. You should prepare to execute your emergency plan. Check that your emergency kit is in place and check the battery-operated devices within. Check to be sure that your shelter and the path to the shelter are accessible. Monitor NOAA Weather Radio or local media outlets for the latest information. Continue about your normal business but stay tuned and alert.

When a tornado watch is issued, think about the drill and check to make sure all your safety supplies are handy. Turn on local TV or radio, or NOAA Weather Radio, and stay alert for warnings. Forget about the old notion of opening windows to equalize pressure; the tornado will blast open the windows for you. If you shop frequently at certain stores, learn where there are bathrooms, storage rooms, or other interior shelter areas away from windows, and the shortest ways to get there. Since we live in an area frequented by tornadoes, when we go anywhere, it's second nature for us to scout out the nearby escapes and shelters. You may not be at home when the warning comes.

Tornado Warning

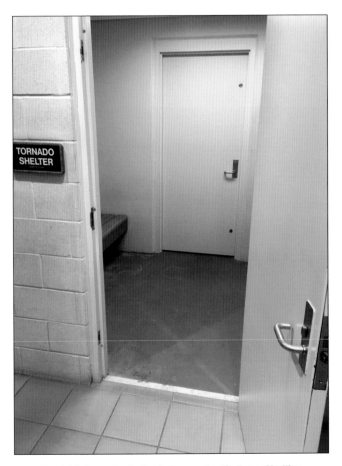

Roadside tornado shelter in Texas. *Credit: Betsy Medling.*

A tornado warning means that a tornado has been spotted, or that Doppler radar indicates a thunderstorm circulation that can (will) spawn a tornado. Take the warning seriously. When a tornado warning is issued for your town or county, take immediate safety precautions. Things are about to get real.

If a tornado warning is issued, or you spot a tornado heading for you, what will you do if you are at home? At work? In your vehicle? Spend a moment to think about it and review it each spring. During a crisis is not the time to think up a plan.

When a warning is issued: A warning means that a tornado has been identified and you are in immediate danger from it.

Survival

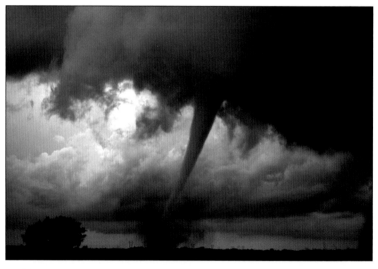

Tornado on the ground near Anadarko, Oklahoma. *Credit: Daphne Zaras.*

Your worst nightmare has come true: you are in a tornado. You've watched the Weather Channel and yelled at the people on television filming the tornado, "get away, idiot, get to shelter, dummy." We've been guilty. We have watched the weather, seen the bad weather is close, and have gone outside to witness the possibility of an oncoming tornado. It's an odd mix of base curiosity and anti-survival logic to purposefully look for a tornado. But it happens. Do as we say, not as we do.

Seek shelter immediately. Every second counts. A shelter should be some place that has sturdy walls, reinforced if possible, preferably in the interior and lowest level of a building. In Tornado Alley, many homes and businesses have dedicated storm cellars or clearly identified tornado shelters.

As the tornado hits, pressure can change so dramatically, your eardrums will pop. The vibrations will be noticeable, the noise even more so.

A safe room is your best bet; unfortunately, the construction of such rooms, especially in older structures or mobile homes, may be impractical or cost prohibitive. However, many rooms in existing structures are safer places than others. If you are in a house or building with a basement, go to the basement. Sounds simple but you'd be surprised

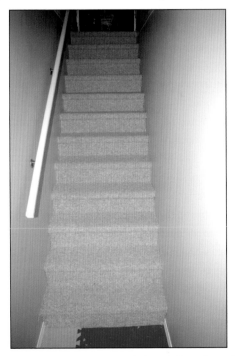

Basements are often the best shelter during a tornado.

how many people don't—through fear or paralysis or the spectacle of it all. If the basement has a small interior room (such as a bathroom or closet) this should be your shelter.

- If your house or building doesn't have a basement, go to the middle of the structure. Small rooms such as bathrooms or closets on the lowest floor are best.
- No room is safe in a mobile home. Evacuate the trailer and go to a designated storm shelter.
- If you find yourself in a home or building with a designated storm shelter, go there immediately. Don't dilly-dally, don't get possessions, just go. Every second counts.
- If you are in charge of safety (workplace, school, etc.), you should immediately enact your tornado safety plan. Your first and main goal is to get everyone in the building to safety.
- When you are in a shelter, assume a safety position. In general, this should be on the floor, on your knees, bent over, with your head against a wall and covered by your arms. Help others get in this position if they need help—children, injured, handicapped, elderly. If you have a pillow or another protective item, place it over your head and neck and secure with your hands.

If you are under tornado threat and you are in a home or building, move quickly to a pre-designated shelter, a basement, or safe-room, and get under a sturdy table or the stairs. Many older homes in Tornado Alley have tornado shelters near the house but building new shelters can be cost-prohibitive compared to safe rooms.

Again, mobile homes, even if you think they are secure or protected, offer little to no protection from tornadoes. There's a reason why after a tornado, the rubble of mobile homes always appears on the television news coverage. Just leave the mobile home and go to the designated storm shelter or the lowest floor of a sturdy building.

If you are out of town, perhaps vacationing, always bring along a NOAA Weather Radio and scope out a place of safety, just in case.

In a house with a basement: Don't get close to windows. If you can, cover the windows. Get you and yours under some kind of sturdy protection, or cover yourself with a mattress or sleeping bag you've strategically placed there in preparation. If there are heavy objects on the floor above you, like a grand piano, don't take shelter directly underneath. The floor can weaken and you'll be under that musical death-drop.

In a house with no basement, a dorm, or an apartment: Avoid windows. Go to the lowest floor, small center room (like a bathroom or closet), under a stairwell, or in an interior hallway with no windows. Crouch as low as possible to the floor, face down, and cover your head with your hands. A bathtub may offer a shell of partial protection. Even in an interior room, you should cover yourself with some sort of thick padding (pillows, mattress, blankets, etc.), to protect against falling debris in case the roof and ceiling fail. A helmet can offer some protection against head injury. If possible, get under a sturdy table, desk or counter. Put as many walls as possible between you and the storm. Stay away from windows.

In an office building, hospital, nursing home or skyscraper: Go directly to an enclosed, windowless area in the center of the building. Get away from glass and on the lowest floor possible. Then, crouch down and cover your head. Interior stairwells are usually good places to take shelter, and if not crowded, allow you to get to a lower level quickly. Stay off the elevators; you could be trapped in them if the power is lost.

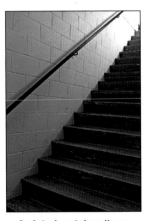

An interior stairwell can serve as shelter.

At school: Follow the drill. Go to the interior hall or room in an orderly way as you are told. Crouch low, head down, and protect the back of your head with your arms. Stay away from windows and large open rooms like gyms and auditoriums.

In a car or truck: You're in your vehicle. Now what? Vehicles are notorious death traps in tornadoes, because they are easily tossed and destroyed. Either leave the vehicle for a sturdy shelter or drive out of the tornado's path. There is no safe option when caught in a tornado in a car, just slightly less dangerous ones. If the tornado is visible, far away, and the traffic is light, you may be able to drive out of its path by moving at right angles to the tornado. Seek shelter in a sturdy building, or underground if possible.

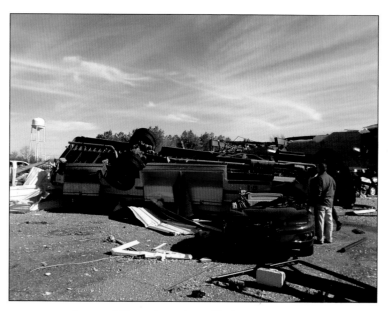

A powerful tornado overturns Oklahoma school bus.
Credit: NWS Jackson, Oklahoma WSFO, NOAA.

Park your car and get out. The idea is to find a deep ditch, some sort of depression to lie down in. It sounds counterintuitive to get out of a perfectly dry, safe, heavy vehicle but here's the truth: your car could easily become a projectile, picked up and slung around by powerful winds. This is more dangerous than lying prone in a muddy ditch. You want to get lower than the level of the roadway. An overpass or bridge might seem safe but a depression or ditch is much safer (traffic hazards, flying debris). So if you are caught in your car before you can safely exit, if you are being pummeled by extreme winds or flying debris and the tornado is upon you, resist the temptation to get out, stay in the car with your seat belt on. Put your head down below the windows; cover your head with your hands and a blanket, coat, or other cushion if possible.

In the open outdoors: If possible, seek shelter in a sturdy building. If not, lie flat and face-down on low ground, protecting the back of your head with your arms. Get as far away from trees and cars as you can; they may be blown onto you in a tornado.

In a shopping mall or large store: Don't panic. Hopefully, when you walked in, you scouted out an exit or a safe place to ride out the storm. Move quickly away from windows to an interior bathroom, storage room or other small, enclosed area. If you see unattended children or people in need, help them get to a safe position or safe room.

In a church or theater: Again, don't panic. Since you'll be in proximity to a large group, scout out multiple exits so you don't get caught up in the mass. Overhead exit signs, side doors. If the tornado is threatening, move quickly but orderly to an interior bathroom or hallway, away from windows. Imagine how much flying glass your typical church will have from stained glass windows. Crouch face-down and protect your head with your arms.

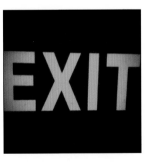

Locate exits in theaters, malls, and other buildings.

If you forget all the other information about surviving tornadoes in this chapter, try to remember these three items:

- This should be your mantra: Do not waste time trying to save personal belongings once you are under the imminent threat of a tornado. Your life and the lives around you are all that matter. Everything else can be replaced.

- Stay low. Winds are slower when lower. Winds increase with height, but the more exposed your body is, the more likely you will be injured by debris.
- Do not go to a group of trees. Tornadoes often contain lightning and that lightning will find a group of trees. By the same token, if there's a single tree in the middle of a field, don't go there either. A single tree is more likely to have a lightning strike than a group of trees.

Tornado Myths and Facts

- **MYTH**: Opening the windows in your house will equalize the pressure when the tornado hits and lessen the damage.
- **FACT**: This is just plain silly and it doesn't work. Your house isn't air-tight and your windows will break from debris and wind-speed so don't waste your time. Tornadoes have too much energy and with your windows closed or open, can tear off your roof or knock down your walls.

- **MYTH**: I live in a big city so we are safe from tornadoes.
- **FACT**: Not true. It doesn't happen often but big cities do get hit and when they do, the destruction is devastating since there is so much concrete and metal to toss around. Dallas, Oklahoma City, Wichita Falls, St. Louis, Miami, and Salt Lake City have all been hit by tornadoes.

- **MYTH**: Mountains never get tornadoes.
- **FACT**: While it's true that higher elevations don't see many tornadoes, it does happen. Utah, New Mexico

and Colorado have all seen tornadoes. Case in point: Cimarron, New Mexico had a tornado tear through town in 1964 and again in 1996, destroying homes and businesses.

- **MYTH**: Cities situated along rivers and by lakes don't get struck by tornadoes because the bodies of water provide protection.
- **FACT**: Decidedly untrue. Water is not a magic boundary against a tornado. History provides many examples of tornadoes that crossed water and still devastated waterside cities.

- **MYTH**: Tornadoes have lifted people up, lifted fragile items up, and miles later, set them down without injury or damage.
- **FACT**: True, in fact. We have lots of anecdotal evidence where people and animals have been transported up to a quarter mile or more without serious injury. But with all the airborne debris, these are the exceptions, rather than the norm.

- **MYTH**: Hiding under a freeway overpass will protect me from a tornado.
- **FACT**: False. While the concrete and rebar in the bridge may offer some protection against flying debris, the overpass also acts as a wind tunnel and may actually serve to collect debris. When you abandon your vehicle at the overpass and climb up the sides, you are doing two things that are hazardous. First, you are blocking the roadway with your vehicle. When the tornado turns all the parked vehicles into a mangled, twisted ball and wedges them under the

overpass, how will emergency vehicles get through? Second, the winds in a tornado tend to be faster with height.

By climbing up off the ground, you place yourself in even greater danger from the tornado and flying debris. When coupled with the accelerated winds due to the wind tunnel (the Venturi Effect) these winds can easily exceed 300 miles per hour. You've felt this before if you've ever stood between two buildings on a windy day and the wind whipped through. Experts claim that you are safer standing in a field than under an overpass. If you realize you won't be able to outrun an approaching tornado, you are much safer to abandon your vehicle, and take shelter in a road-side ditch or other low spot.

- **MYTH**: I can outrun a tornado in my vehicle.
- **FACT:** You might, but unless you can predict a tornado's path, and experts still cannot do that, it's a dicey move. Besides, tornadoes can travel at 70 miles per hour or more. They often shift directions erratically, without warning. You are better off abandoning your vehicle and seeking shelter immediately.

- **MYTH**: While there is no such thing as a Category 6 hurricane (the Saffir-Simpson Hurricane only goes to Category 5), there can be an F6 tornado.
- **FACT:** Technically, yes. Practically, no. The Fujita Tornado Damage Intensity Scale actually goes up to F12. The F12 level only begins at wind speeds exceeding Mach 1.0 (or around 738 miles per hour at -3°C), so the probability of a tornado having winds of this speed is infinitesimally small. Could a tornado

be an F6? Yes; however, the Fujita scale is based on wind speeds that are estimated from the damage the tornado produced (because no one has been able to stick an anemometer into a tornado to measure the actual wind speeds). Since the winds of an F5 tornado (up to 319 miles per hour) are sufficient to completely destroy just about everything in its path, an F6 really wouldn't do much more damage than that, and therefore could not be definitively labeled as an F6.

- **MYTH**: Tornadoes are more likely to hit a mobile home park.
- **FACT:** Not so. It just seems that way for two reasons. First, mobile home parks are a ubiquitous part of our landscape. There are tens of thousands of mobile homes in Tornado Alley, so there is a good likelihood that some of them will be in the path of a tornado. Unfortunately, the second factor is that mobile homes

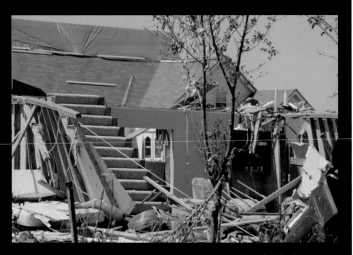

Tornado destruction in Moore, Oklahoma. *Credit: Pixabay.*

offer little to no protection against even the weakest tornadoes, so when a tornado does strike a mobile home park, the damage is more likely to be significant. Winds that would only lift some shingles on a frame house can easily flip a mobile home.

- **MYTH**: Strong, sturdy brick or stone buildings will protect me from a tornado.
- **FACT:** While such buildings will provide more protection in a tornado than a mobile home or timber frame structure, the winds of a tornado can easily launch a 2x4 through a brick wall, and can cause even the sturdiest of buildings to experience roof or wall failure. The safest location in your home is wherever you have a small, windowless, interior room on the lowest level of your house.

- **MYTH**: A tornado is not coming directly at me; I am safe.
- **FACT:** Tornados often act erratically, often changing directions quickly. Sturdy shelter is the only safe place to be during a tornado. Although it may be tempting to follow a tornado to get a cool photo, please leave the tornado chasing to trained meteorologists.

- **MYTH:** Tornadoes never strike the same location twice.
- **FACT:** Not true at all. The town of Cordell, Kansas had a tornado hit on May 20 three years in a row (1916, 1917, and 1918). In Guy, Arkansas, three tornadoes hit the same church on the same day. One hit in Cimarron, New Mexico in 1964 and 1996.

- **MYTH:** The shape and size of the tornado determines its strength.
- **FACT:** Tornadoes come in all shapes and sizes and one should not depend on their size or shape to determine strength. The only way to determine the strength of the tornado is through damage assessments conducted by the National Weather Service or by taking a direct measurement of wind. During damage assessments, National Weather Service employees look for clues that will indicate how strong the winds were. The wind estimate is then related to the Enhanced-Fujita tornado scale and a tornado intensity level will be assigned. Tornadoes are rated on a scale from EF0 to EF5, with EF5 being the strongest. Merely by looking at the tornado's shape does not tell the whole story. The visible funnel is created by cloud condensation or dirt and debris. Conditions that create the visible funnel will change each time a tornado develops . . . and therefore one cannot use this method reliably.

- **MYTH:** The number of tornadoes per year has been increasing due to more favorable weather conditions.
- **FACT:** Scientists discount the idea that climate change or global warming has affected the number of documented tornadoes in America. The number of documented tornadoes in the US has indeed increased since the early 1900s but this increase is mostly likely due to the general increase in the population. We have more trained storm spotters, better radar detection technology, and better follow-up damage surveys. Tornadoes have not become more common due to more favorable weather conditions.

Aftermath

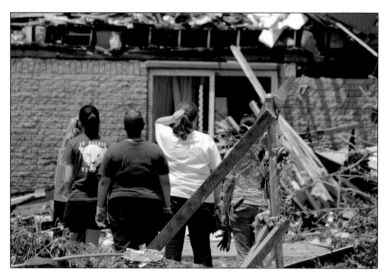

Assessing tornado damage in Moore, Oklahoma. *Credit: Pixabay.*

The tornado will have come and gone in a terrifying moment, a few seconds to a few minutes. The worst has passed but you're not out of danger yet. First, you need to assess the situation. Are you or any people around you injured? Trapped? If you are trapped, don't panic. You may be in a dangerous situation, and panicked movements may cause further injury. Call for help. If you have a cell phone, it may still work but the landlines might be down. If there are few visible reference points remaining above ground, attempt to mark existing landmarks with addresses so rescue personnel can navigate and respond effectively. When trained emergency responders arrive, comply with their directives.

If you are not trapped and there are injured around you, go into first-aid mode. If you're at home or in a shelter, you should have a first-aid kit available. Only once they are stable, do you call for rescue and alert the authorities.

Assess the structure you are in. Does it seem stable? Are there parts of the wall or roof falling down or look like they might? Often, electrical power lines are downed and gas lines may be leaking. Broken tree limbs, glass, and other debris may litter the ground, creating further hazards. You also must worry about structural integrity of the shelter or building. If the building is damaged, if there are electrical sparks visible, or the smell of gas or chemical fumes is present, carefully leave the building. If possible, turn off the gas, electricity, and water to the building. Do not return until you are advised by authorities that the structure is safe. If so, get you and others out as best you can.

Since tornadoes are usually thunderstorm-borne, there is usually a heavy downpour of rain after the tornado passes, even though there may be no rain present during the actual tornado. Flooding is a very real possibility. There may also be damaging hail.

If the building is not damaged and there is no evidence of utility damage, inspect the building for any flammable liquid spills—bleaches, cleaning fluid, etc., and immediately clean them up.

Tornadoes are categorized as levels 0 to 5 by the Enhanced Fujita Scale, which is based on wind speeds and the amount of damage caused:

- **F0 Light:** Winds 40 to 72 miles per hour; smaller trees uprooted or branches broken, mild structural damage.

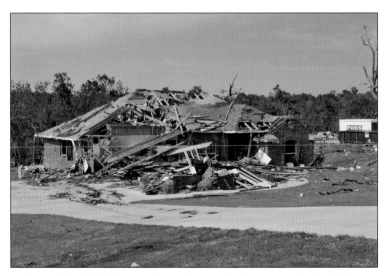

Destruction of a brick home in the aftermath of a tornado. *Credit: Pixabay.*

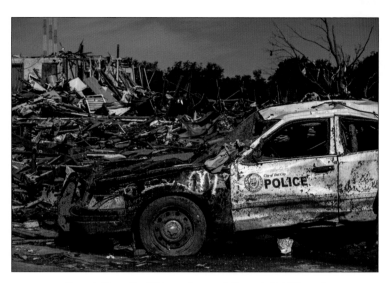

Devastation after F5 tornado swept through Del City and surrounding areas of Oklahoma. *Credit: Pixabay.*

- **F1 Moderate:** Winds 73 to 112 miles per hour; broken windows, small tree trunks broken, overturned mobile homes, destruction of carports or toolsheds, roof tiles missing.
- **F2 Considerable:** Winds 113 to 157 miles per hour; mobile homes destroyed, major structural damage to frame homes due to flying debris, some large trees snapped in half or uprooted.
- **F3 Severe:** Winds 158 to 206 miles per hour; roofs torn from homes, small frame homes destroyed, most trees snapped and uprooted.
- **F4 Devastating:** Winds 207 to 260 miles per hour; strong-structured buildings damaged or destroyed or lifted from foundations, cars lifted and blown away, even large debris airborne.
- **F5 Incredible:** Winds 261 to 318 miles per hour; larger buildings lifted from foundations, trees snapped, uprooted and debarked, objects weighing more than a ton become airborne missiles.

CHAPTER FOUR

TSUNAMIS

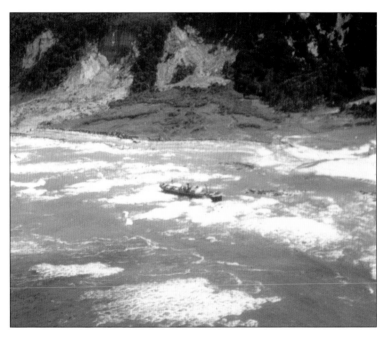

Tsunami hitting on Isla Mocha in 1960. *Credit: Pierre St. Amand.*

Tsunamis are the most infrequent of all the weather disasters covered in this book, but each tsunami event has the potential to be utterly devastating. Until the 2004 Indian Ocean Tsunami, we, like many other

Americans, knew little about tsunamis and erroneously thought them so rare that they held a mythic quality.

The Indian Ocean Tsunami of December 26, 2004 woke the world up to the power and devastation of a tsunami. At 7:58 a.m., a powerful 9.3 magnitude earthquake, the third most powerful ever recorded, occurred in the Indian Ocean just west of Sumatra. The quake lasted ten minutes (the longest duration ever recorded), generating tsunami waves in every direction. The waves hit the coast of Sumatra quickly and first, with eighty- to one-hundred-foot waves smashing into communities, obliterating anything in the path. An estimated 150,000 lives were lost and a half-million people left homeless.

Thailand was the next target of the tsunami as it moved eastward across the Indian Ocean. An estimated ten thousand perished there. An hour and a half after the initial earthquake, Sri Lanka was hit; later, the tsunami struck India, South Africa, and other countries, leaving destruction and death. All told, 190,000 to 225,000 people died, with another forty to fifty thousand missing and presumed dead.

So, what is a tsunami? According to the International Tsunami Information Center, a tsunami is a series of large waves of extremely long wavelength and period usually generated by a violent, impulsive undersea disturbance or activity near the coast or in the ocean. When a sudden displacement of a large volume of water occurs, or if the sea floor is suddenly raised or dropped by an earthquake, big tsunami waves can be formed. The waves travel out of the area of origin and can be extremely dangerous and damaging when they reach the shore.

Tsunamis move great lengths with tremendous power. Tsunamis are not tidal waves despite the fact that this moniker is often associated with them. Tsunamis (pronounced soo-ná-mees) are a series of powerful waves initiated by an underwater disruption such as an earthquake, landslide, volcanic eruption, explosion, or even meteorite. From the area where the tsunami originates, waves travel outward in all directions.

Tsunamis amazingly move hundreds of miles per hour in the open ocean, up to 500 miles per hour. In the deep ocean, tsunami waves may appear only a foot or so high. A tsunami travels at a speed that is related to the water depth—hence, as the water depth decreases, the tsunami slows. The tsunami's energy flux, which is dependent on both its wave speed and wave height, remains nearly constant.

As the wave approaches the shoreline and enters shallower water, it slows down and begins to grow in energy and height. The tops of the waves move faster than their bottoms do, which causes them to rise precipitously. Consequently, as the tsunami's speed diminishes, its height grows. This is called shoaling. Because of this shoaling effect, a tsunami that is unnoticeable at sea may grow to be several feet or more in height near the coast.

So, as a tsunami wave approaches shallow water, the wave slows, causing the quicker-traveling water to pull up, which in turn extends the wave vertically. When the waves reach the shore, the waves build, and these waves can reach one hundred feet (although most of the time, the wave will be much less in height) with multiple waves occurring in succession. The topography of the coastline and the ocean floor will influence the size of the wave. There will likely be more than one wave and the succeeding ones will often be larger than the one before. That is why a small tsunami at one beach can be a giant wave a few miles away.

For tsunamis that are generated by underwater earthquakes, the amplitude of the tsunami is determined by the amount by which the sea-floor is displaced. Similarly, the wavelength and period of the tsunami are determined by the size and shape of the underwater disturbance. As well as travelling at high speeds, tsunamis can also travel large distances without losing much energy. As the tsunami moves across the ocean, the wave-crests can undergo refraction (bending), which is caused by segments of the wave moving at different speeds as the water depth along the wave crest varies. If you are in deep water, it is unlikely you'd even notice a tsunami passing your boat or ship.

Tsunami waves come in a series. The distance between crests often exceeds sixty miles. In deep water they may be only a few inches high at the surface and will pass beneath a boat undetected. When the waves approach shallow water, they slow down and build in height. A tsunami can hit shore as a huge wave a hundred feet high. Most of the time, they arrive as a deadly, turbulent surge of whitewater.

This list comprises the ten worst tsunamis in history based on fatalities since the year 1700.

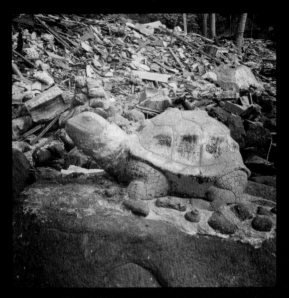

Tsunami destruction in Phuket, Thailand. *Credit: Pixabay.*

1. Indian Ocean Tsunami
2004, 9.1–9.3 in magnitude, killed more than 283,000 people and reached fourteen countries.

2. Messina, Italy Earthquake and Tsunami
December 28, 1908, earthquake, 7.1, 100,000 to 200,000 killed.

3. Portugal-Morocco Tsunami
1755, Lisbon, Portugal, 9.0 earthquake, 60,000 to 100,000 people.

4. Tsunami in South Chinese Sea, 1782
Earthquake, 40,000 people killed.

5. Krakatoa, Indonesia Tsunami

August 26–27 in 1883, legendary series of massive explosions, the eruption of Krakatoa. The sounds produced by this volcanic eruption are considered to be the loudest sounds ever heard in modern history. Tsunamis killed over 40,000 people.

6. Tokaido-Nankaido, Japan Tsunami

1707, earthquake, 8.4 magnitude 1707, 30,000 people died.

7. Sanriku, Japan Tsunami

1896, 8.5 in magnitude, 27,000 deaths.

8. Southern Chile Earthquake and Tsunami

May, 1960, possibly the largest earthquake (9.5) in recorded history occurred on May 22, 1960 off the coast of Chile. The ensuing tsunamis caused up to 6,000 deaths.

9. Tohoku Earthquake and Tsunami

2011 earthquake of Tohoku registered a 9.0 magnitude, 15,884 people lost their lives in the resulting tsunami; also caused the nuclear disaster of Fukushima.

10. Ryukyu Islands Tsunami

1771, earthquake 7.4 in magnitude. The tsunami claimed a third of the population (over 12,000 lives).

Since 1975, there have been forty-two deadly tsunamis, and 76 percent of those occurred in the Pacific and its related seas. Over history, 1610 BCE to 2016, there have been 1,235 confirmed tsunamis, of which 249 have been deadly. Eighty-seven percent of the tsunamis were caused by earthquakes. Tsunamis are blind to predictions, politics or borders, wreaking havoc and crossing ocean basins with deadly waves that can reach several stories in height. Tsunamis can flood as far as ten miles inland.

Things to Know About Tsunamis:

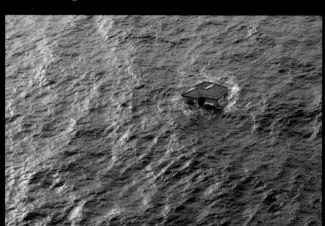

A house adrift during the 2011 tsunami in Sendai, Japan.
Credit: Mass Communication Specialist 3rd Class Dylan McCord

1. About 80 percent of tsunamis happen within the Pacific Ocean's "Ring of Fire."
2. The first wave of a tsunami is usually not the strongest, successive waves get bigger and stronger.
3. Tsunamis can travel at speeds of about five hundred miles or 805 kilometers an hour, almost as fast as a jet plane.
4. The states in the US at greatest risk for tsunamis are Hawaii, Alaska, Washington, Oregon, and California.
5. If caught by a tsunami wave, it is better not to swim, but rather to grab a floating object and allow the current to carry you.
6. Tsunamis retain their energy, meaning they can travel across entire oceans with limited energy loss.
7. Tsunami means "harbor wave" in Japanese (*tsu* = harbor + *nami* = wave), reflecting Japan's tsunami-prone history.

8. Scientists can accurately estimate the time when a tsunami will arrive almost anywhere around the world based on calculations using the depth of the water, distances from one place to another, and the time that the earthquake or other event occurred.

9. Hawaii is always at great risk for a tsunami—they get about one per year and a severe one every seven years. The biggest tsunami that occurred in Hawaii happened in 1946. The coast of Hilo Island was hit with thirty-foot waves at 500 miles per hour.

10. In 2004, the Indian Ocean tsunami was caused by an earthquake with the energy of 23,000 atomic bombs. After the earthquake, killer waves radiating from the epicenter slammed into the coastline of eleven countries. The final death toll was 283,000.

The best defense against any tsunami is early warning that allows people to seek higher ground. The Pacific Tsunami Warning System, a coalition of twenty-six nations headquartered in Hawaii, maintains a

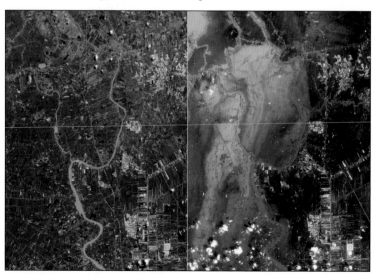

Ayutthaya, Thailand before and after a tsunami. *Credit: Pixabay.*

web of seismic equipment and water level gauges to identify tsunamis at sea. Similar systems are proposed to protect coastal areas worldwide.

Improved Warning Systems: The National Oceanic and Atmospheric Administration (NOAA) bears the primary responsibility of providing tsunami warnings. NOAA established the Seismic Sea Wave Warning System in Hawaii, the forerunner of the current Pacific Tsunami Warning System, in 1949. NOAA created the West Coast/Alaska Tsunami Warning Center (WC / ATWC) in Palmer, Alaska, in 1967 as a direct result of the great 9.2 Alaska earthquake of 1964. Today, the WC/ATWC continues to issue tsunami warnings for Alaska, British Columbia, Washington, Oregon, and California. TsunamiReady works with community leaders and emergency administrators to develop plans that include evacuation routes and redundant systems of alerting the public. Visit www.tsunamiready.noaa.gov/ts-communities.htm for a list of TsunamiReady sites.

Tide Gauges: Tide gauges measure the height of the sea-surface and are primarily used for measuring tide levels. Most of the tide gauges operated by the Bureau of Meteorology's National Tidal Centre are SEAFRAME stations (Sea Level Fine Resolution Acoustic Measuring Equipment).

Satellites: Satellite altimeters measure the height of the ocean surface directly by use of electromagnetic pulses.

The DART System: In 1995, the National Oceanic and Atmospheric Administration (NOAA) began developing the Deep-ocean Assessment and Reporting of Tsunamis (DART) system. An array of stations is currently deployed in the Pacific Ocean. These stations give detailed information about tsunamis while they are still far off shore. The system has considerably improved the forecasting and warning of tsunamis in the Pacific.

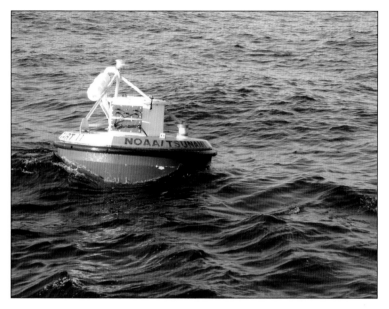

Tsunami DART system. *Credit: Allen Shimada, NOAA.*

Preparation

Tsunamis are a true force of nature. They can hoist boulders and sweep buildings right off their foundations. They destroy coastal communities and kill thousands of people. Should you worry? Did you know that over one third of the world's population lives within sixty miles of the ocean? Forty percent of the population of the United States lives in counties directly on the shoreline, and the coast is only expected to become more crowded. That's why you need to be prepared in case one of these rare but devastating waves comes to a beach near you.

Three things:

1. Determine if you are at risk from tsunamis.
2. Seek knowledge. Become tsunami savvy.
3. Act quickly. Be ready to launch a plan of action without hesitation.

I know this advice sounds great in theory, but in practice, seems impractical. If you ever find yourself in a tsunami-alert situation, you'll wish you had done this: practiced an emergency drill with your family. This might be the difference, in a crisis, between living and dying. Make sure each member of your family knows his/her role in the emergency plan, where to go, and what to take. In fact, if you are serious about it, you need to prepare a "tsunami kit," which includes first aid, the essentials, plans to evacuate family and pets, various evacuation routes and meeting places, and provisions to last at least three days for each family member.

Let's assume you are serious about preparation. If you prepare properly, you can put yourself and your family out of harm's way of a deadly tsunami.

First, know the tsunami evacuation zone. Know your community's disaster plans. Map out and practice an evacuation route, and have a kit ready for emergencies. Sounds easy right?

Here's how to do all that:

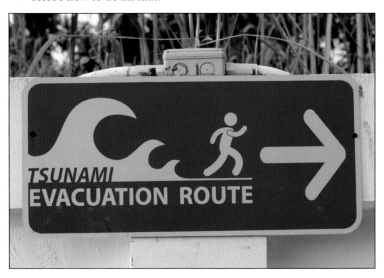

Make note of tsunami evacuation routes. *Credit: Pixabay.*

Develop an evacuation plan. Yes, this seems like a perfectly reasonable thing to do, one of those logical things we never actually get around to doing. You can't wait until the radio informs you that your community is under tsunami watch or warning to prepare your evacuation plan. In advance, think about where you and your family might be in the community—work, school, home—when a tsunami might hit. Develop multiple plans that allow for the evacuation from wherever you and yours might be. If your community has an evacuation plan, learn it. If they do not, why not be involved and help develop it?

Lack of evacuation plans and local warning systems put you, your family, and your entire community at increased risk for injury or death during and after a tsunami. These are the steps to making a successful evacuation plan:

- Discuss with family and colleagues the various options for evacuation. Know, for example, where you might reunite with your loved ones should a tsunami hit.
- Conduct practice drills to ensure that all members of the community are clear about what they need to do and where they need to go during a safety evacuation.
- Include a plan that can ensure a head count of every single member of the community; ensure that assistance for disabled or ill persons can be provided.
- Ensure that warning and evacuation signals are understood by the community in advance.
- Remember to provide multiple safety routes since an earthquake could destroy roads and other infrastructure, preventing exit using some routes.
- Consider what types of sheltered areas might exist in the evacuation zones; do such shelters need to be built in advance? Could these shelters be used to hold fresh water and food?

Know if tsunamis have struck your coastal region in the past. Do your own sleuthing and do some library research or ask at the local government office. FEMA has a website enabling online flood risk searches.

Know the height of your street above sea level and the distance of your street from the coast or other high-risk waters. Evacuation orders may be based on these numbers. Also, find out the height above sea level and the distance from the coast of outbuildings that house animals, as well as pastures or corrals.

Plan evacuation routes from your home, school, workplace, or any other place you could be where tsunamis present a risk. If possible, pick areas one hundred feet above sea level or go as far as two miles inland, away from the coastline. If you cannot get this high or far, go as high or far as you can. Every foot inland or upward may make a difference. You should be able to reach your safe location on foot within fifteen minutes. After a disaster, roads may become impassable or blocked.

Be prepared to evacuate by foot if necessary. Footpaths typically lead uphill and inland, while many roads parallel coastlines. Follow posted tsunami evacuation routes; these will lead to safety. Local emergency management officials can advise you on the best route to safety and likely shelter locations.

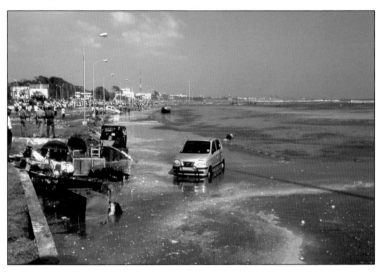

Beach flood after a tsunami in Chennai on Bay of Bengal in eastern India.
*Credit: Kotoviski on sv.wikipedia (Fotograferad av Henryk Kotowski.) [GFDL
(http-_www.gnu.org_copyleft_fdl.html)*

If your children's school is in an identified inundation zone (that area that expects to receive a large amount of flood water), find out what the school evacuation plan is. Find out if the plan requires you to pick your children up from school or from another location.

Practice your evacuation routes. Familiarity with these routes may save your life, but it does no good if you are the only one in your family to know the routes. Be able to follow your escape route at night and during inclement weather. Practicing your plan makes the appropriate response more of a reaction, requiring less thinking during an actual emergency.

Use a NOAA Weather Radio or stay tuned to a local radio or television station to keep informed of local watches and warnings.

Talk to your insurance agent. Homeowners' policies do not cover flooding from a tsunami. Ask about the National Flood Insurance Program (NFIP) (www.fema.gov/nfip). NFIP covers tsunami damage, but your community must participate in the program. We have more about how to file insurance in the Aftermath section of this chapter.

If you are visiting an area at risk from tsunamis, check with the hotel, motel, or campground operators for tsunami evacuation information and find out what the warning system is for tsunamis. It is important to know designated escape routes before a warning is issued.

Make sure you have access to NOAA radio broadcasts to stay informed of ever-changing conditions:

- Find an online NOAA radio station: (http://www.nws .noaa.gov/nwr/coverage/station_listing.html).
- Search for a NOAA radio app.
- If you do live in a coastal area, elevate your home to help reduce damage. Most tsunami waves are less than ten feet (three meters).
- Take precautions to prevent flooding (sandbags are a common preventive measure).
- Have an engineer check your home and advise about how to make it more resistant to tsunami water. There may be ways to divert waves away from your property. Improperly built walls could make your situation worse.

You can't take a lot with you in the event of a tsunami. You'll want to take your computer, but it stays. There is no room. You can do several things to save yourself the futility of losing your laptop. Back files up with redundancy. Email files to yourself. Save to the cloud. Save to various hard-drives and store them at your parents' house, your work, a safe deposit box. Yeah, it hurts to leave the laptop behind, but your data are more important.

TIP: Have large Ziplock-type bags at the house, and if you have time, you can stuff your laptop into the bag and store the laptop high up in a closet.

TSUNAMI PREPAREDNESS KIT

Being prepared means being equipped with the proper supplies you may need in the event of an emergency or disaster. Store your "tsunami kit" in an obvious, easy to reach place that everyone in the family can access. Store the supplies in an easy-to-carry emergency waterproof bag that you can use at home or take with you in case you must evacuate. Depending on your family needs and the ages of family members, you might prefer to create a personal safety pack for each family member. Individual packs can include more personalized supplies like medications, personal information, extra glasses, personal needs, etc. These packs can be stored individually or compiled into one larger storage bag.

At a minimum, you should have the basic supplies listed below:

- Water: one gallon per person per day (three-day supply for evacuation, two-week supply for home).
- Food: non-perishable, easy-to-prepare items (three-day supply for evacuation, day-week supply for home).
- Battery-powered or hand-crank radio (NOAA Weather Radio, if possible. Batteries can get wet and while the hand-crank radio seems like a pain, it's not that hard to use. You could always have both.
- Extra batteries.
- First-aid kit.

- Medications (seven-day supply) and medical items.
- Multi-purpose tool or pocket knife.
- Sanitation and personal hygiene items (soap, toothpaste, toothbrush, hand wipes, etc.).
- Several plastic, Ziplock baggies of varying sizes (you can put your phone in one, your papers in another, etc.).
- Copies of personal documents (medication list and pertinent medical information, proof of address, deed/lease to home, passports, birth certificates, photo identification, insurance policies, bank account, and credit card information).
- Cell phone with charger. (Consider adding an instant phone charger, which costs around ten bucks, because it's likely that power outages will occur after the tsunami hits.)
- Family and emergency contact information, including a written list of phone numbers.
- Extra cash and change, as ATMs may not be working.
- Emergency blanket. (We recommend buying several small emergency thermal blankets, like the compact silver ones that come in a small package. They aren't much bigger than a wallet and provide warmth.)
- Map of the surrounding area, including an agreed-upon meeting spot in case of separation and the nearest safe shelter.
- Shoes. (We're fisherman and have used lightweight sandals designed for wading. They are lightweight, have grip, and are ideal for the kit. Flip-flops won't work in flood conditions. They will come off, leaving your feet exposed to underwater dangers. Shoes designed for wading will keep you better protected. A pair of old canvas slip-on tennis shoes with a thick rubber sole would work too.)

Other items to consider adding to your preparedness kit when trying to meet the needs of all family members and especially if you want to create a mega pack.

- Additional medical supplies (hearing aids with extra batteries, glasses, contact lenses, contact solution, syringes, etc.).
- Baby supplies (bottles, formula, baby food, diapers).
- Games and activities for children.
- Change of clothing and undergarments.
- Pet supplies (see sidebar for details).
- Two-way radios.
- Extra set of car keys and house keys.
- Manual can opener.
- Moist towelettes, garbage bags and plastic ties for personal sanitation.
- Feminine products.
- Plastic sheeting and duct tape to shelter-in-place.
- Wrench or pliers to turn off utilities.
- Reference materials for first aid, book or photocopies.
- Rain gear.
- Tent.
- Compass.
- Paracord (rope).
- Bleach, disinfectant, and antibacterial wipes. (Use bleach as a disinfectant, nine parts water, one part bleach and if necessary, to treat water by using sixteen drops of regular household liquid bleach per gallon of water. Do not use scented, color safe, or bleaches with added cleaners.)
- Medicine dropper.
- Paper towels.
- Paper and pencil.
- Matches in waterproof container.
- Fire extinguisher.
- Traveler's checks.
- Camp-style mess kit, paper plates, cups, utensils.

Clothing and Bedding

Preparing clothing and bedding is especially important if you live in a cold climate. You'll want to be as warm as possible when temperatures drop and potential power outages occur. Compile a warm set of clothing and pair of shoes for each person in your family. Revisit your supply at least once a year to account for growing children and family changes. Items to include:

- Coat.
- Long pants.
- Long-sleeved shirt.
- Silk or insulated pant/top liners.
- Sturdy shoes.
- Wicking socks.
- Hat and gloves.
- Sleeping bag or warm blanket for each person.
- Hand and boot warmers, emergency warming blankets.

Preparedness Kit for Pets:

- Food, bottled water, and medication for at least seven days (rotate out with new every few months to keep your kit fresh).
- Photocopies of medical/immunization records and current photo of your pet in case you get separated.
- Extra leash, collar, or harness.
- Feeding/drinking dish.
- Plastic bags for cleanup.

(Continued)

- Aluminum roasting pans for use as litter trays, litter, or paper toweling.
- Blanket (comfort or to wrap up a scared pet).
- Liquid dish soap, disinfectant, or antibacterial wipes.
- Evac-Sack or pillowcase, especially for cats. (Evac-Sacks are the way to go for any small animal.)
- Play and/or chew toys.
- Cage liner.

Try to assemble your preparedness kit well in advance of an emergency. You may have to evacuate at a moment's notice and take essentials with you. You will probably not have time to search for the supplies you need or shop for them. Teach family members how to use text messaging (or SMS). Text messages can often get around network disruptions when a phone call might not be able to get through. Subscribe to alert services. Receive alerts via Twitter, text, or email.

Rally the community behind a rehabilitation plan. If local authorities have not put action plans into place, suggest that they do so or form a community action group to consider a post-tsunami plan. Things that can help survival post-tsunami include:

- Establish an advance stash of fresh water. Whether bottled water or filtered water, an emergency water supply should be in place in your community.
- Open up undamaged homes and buildings to others. Locate those places on higher ground and ensure usage during emergency. Help those in distress and provide them with shelter.
- Ensure the community has power generators to enable cooking, maintenance of hygiene, and return of basic health and transportation services.
- Run emergency shelters and food distribution.

- Get health care into action immediately.
- Quell fires and gas ruptures.

Escape Routes and Meeting Place

Draw a floor plan of your home. Use a blank sheet of paper for each floor. Mark two escape routes from each room. Make sure children understand the drawings. Post a copy of the drawings at eye level in each child's room. If one option of your escape route is to go to the roof of your house, how will each of you get up to the roof? Do you have ladders? Are they uselessly stored in a shed in the backyard? You might look at some ladder options for emergencies. And make certain everyone in your family knows how to deploy and use the ladder.

It's a good idea to establish a meeting place for your family in the event that you have enough time before the tsunami hits. Establish a meeting place for after the tsunami event is over since you all might not be together when the waves hit. Hopefully, the meeting place after will be at your house.

Plan for Various Locations

Individuals and households should consider the locations they frequent; find out what emergency plans are in place for these locations. Once you know that, you can customize your personal and household plans based on what your household members would do if an emergency occurred while they were at that location. Examples of locations to consider and plan for include:

- Home.
- Workplace.
- Vehicles.
- Regular methods of transportation, such as trains or urban commuter transit or your car's normal routes.
- School.
- Places of worship.
- Sports arenas and playing fields.

- Entertainment locations, such as theaters.
- Shopping areas, such as malls and retail centers.
- Tourist and travel locations, such as hotels (especially if you are a tourist).

Developing plans for different locations will require getting key information about the organization or building managers' plans for the locations. If plans are not available, this may involve working with the building manager or other members of the organization to develop or expand plans. Information that should be considered includes:

- How you and other occupants will get local alert or warnings while you are there.
- Building location alarm or alert systems.
- Building occupant evacuation plans including alternate exits.
- Building or organization plans for sheltering occupants in an emergency.
- Key supplies you/household members and others would need for temporary sheltering.

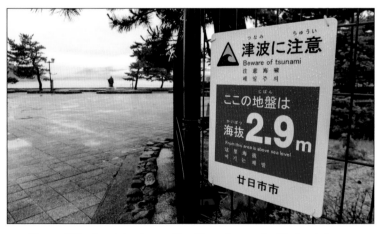

Shore of Miyajima Island, near Hiroshima, Japan. *Credit: Joe deSousa.*

Survival

There are four levels of tsunami alerts issued for United States, Canadian, and British Virgin Islands coastal communities: warning, advisory, watch, and information statement. Each has a distinct meaning relating to local emergency response. Recommended protective actions vary within areas under warnings and advisories. Be alert to and follow instructions from local emergency officials because they may have more detailed or specific information.

Alert Level	Potential Hazard(s)	Action
Warning	Dangerous coastal flooding and powerful currents	Move to high ground or inland
Advisory	Strong currents and waves dangerous to those in or very near water	Stay out of water, away from beaches and waterways
Watch	Not yet known	Stay tuned for more information Be prepared to act
Information Statement	No threat or very distant event for which hazard has not been determined	No action suggested at this time

Tsunami Warning: From the NOAA: "A tsunami warning is issued when a tsunami with the potential to generate widespread inundation is imminent, expected, or occurring. Warnings alert the public that dangerous coastal flooding accompanied by powerful currents is possible and may continue for several hours after initial arrival. Warnings alert emergency management officials to take action for the entire tsunami hazard zone. Appropriate actions to be taken by local officials may include the evacuation of low-lying coastal areas, and the repositioning of ships to deep waters when there is time to safely do so. Warnings may be updated, adjusted geographically, downgraded, or canceled based on updated information and analysis."

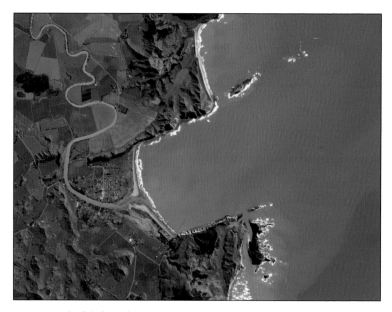

Aerial view of emergency tsunami watch after 7.1 quake;
Tolaga Bay, New Zealand. *Credit: Planet Labs.*

Tsunami Advisory: From the NOAA: "A tsunami advisory is issued when a tsunami with the potential to generate strong currents or waves dangerous to those in or very near the water is imminent, expected, or occurring. The threat may continue for several hours after initial arrival, but significant inundation is not expected for areas under an advisory. Appropriate actions to be taken by local officials may include closing beaches, evacuating harbors and marinas, and the repositioning of ships to deep waters when there is time to safely do so. Advisories may be updated, adjusted geographically, upgraded to a warning, or cancelled based on updated information and analysis."

Tsunami Watch: From the NOAA: "A tsunami watch is issued when a tsunami may later impact the watch area. The watch may be upgraded to a warning or advisory or canceled based on updated information and analysis. Emergency management officials and the public should prepare to take action."

Tsunami Information Statement: From the NOAA: "A tsunami information statement is issued when an earthquake or tsunami has occurred of interest to the message recipients. In most cases, information statements are issued to indicate there is no threat of a destructive basin-wide tsunami and to prevent unnecessary evacuations. Information statements for distant events requiring evaluation may be upgraded to a warning, advisory, or watch based on updated information and analysis. A cancellation is issued after an evaluation of water-level data confirms that a destructive tsunami will not impact an area under a warning, advisory, or watch or that a tsunami has diminished to a level where additional damage is not expected."

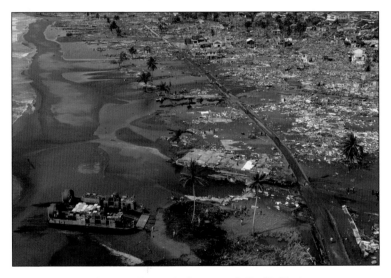

The flooded aftermath of a tsunami. *Credit: Pixabay.*

International Tsunami Messages

International tsunami messages are issued by the Pacific Tsunami Warning Center to international partners in the Pacific and Caribbean and Adjacent Regions for guidance only in support of the UNESCO/IOC Pacific Tsunami Warning and Mitigation System and the Tsunami and Other Coastal Hazards Warning System for the Caribbean and

Adjacent Regions. There are two types of international tsunami messages: tsunami threat messages and information statements. These messages do not include alerts. The primary purpose of these messages is to help national authorities understand the threat to their coasts so they can determine which alerts to issue for their coastlines, if any.

Alert Level	Potential Hazard(s)	Action
Threat	Dangerous coastal flooding and/or powerful currents	Get more information, follow instructions from national and local authorities
Information Statement	Minor waves at most	No action suggested

Tsunami Threat Message: A tsunami threat message is issued to national authorities when a tsunami may affect their coasts. It describes the tsunami threats according to the potential hazard and impact to people, structures, and ecosystems on land or in nearshore marine environments. National authorities will determine the appropriate level of alert for each country and may issue additional or more refined information and instructions. Threat messages may be updated based on new information, data and analysis.

A final tsunami threat message is issued when the Pacific Tsunami Warning Center determines there is no further threat.

Tsunami Information Statement: A tsunami information statement is issued to national authorities when an earthquake or tsunami has occurred of interest to the message recipients. In most cases, information statements are issued to indicate there is no threat of a tsunami and to prevent unnecessary evacuations. Information statements may be upgraded to tsunami threats based on updated information and analysis.

Tsunami Warning Signs and What to Do:

First clue: An earthquake. If your community is coastal, it is likely tied into any of several tsunami detection/warning systems. If you are in an earthquake on the coast, pay attention, and if the earthquake lasts a good while, say thirty seconds, go into tsunami alert mode.

Second clue: If you are on a boat, sitting on a dock in the bay or drinking daiquiris at a tiki bar on the beach, and you are in an earthquake or receive news that there was a major earthquake at sea, quickly assess the situation and get to higher land. Don't wait. Think elevation gain, not just moving away from the coast. Tsunamis travel far inland on flat land.

Third clue: Receding water. A predictor of a tsunami is that the water in the bay/harbor suddenly recedes often leaving an exposed sea bottom. If you watch the YouTube videos of tsunamis from 2004 to present, one commonality is that when the water recedes, people are fascinated and stick around, and then the tsunami is upon them and it's too late. If the water recedes dramatically, leave immediately!

If you are on a boat and this occurs, get out and get to safety, or if you can still maneuver the boat, take the boat out to deeper water. Naturally, the latter action assumes more risk. But staying on the boat and facing the impending series of powerful waves is riskier. If you are prepared, you will have local charts so you can know water depths outside the harbor. How deep is safe? Six hundred feet at the minimum, and twelve hundred feet preferably.

Fourth clue: Earthquakes and tsunamis release unbelievable amounts of energy. Some additional natural signs that a tsunami may be imminent are odd sounds, weird vibrations, and unusual water behavior. Sometimes before a tsunami hits, the water gets frothy with bubbles and exhibits strange conflicting currents wherein moored vessels bob or sway violently.

Fifth clue: Animals have a sense for changes in nature, and they display it if you watch closely. If your pets act abnormally, perk up.

Sixth and final clue: Local, government, and international organizations are better than ever at warning of possible tsunamis. Pay attention. Inform yourself in advance of how the local authorities plan to make warnings so that you do not mistake or ignore the warning when it comes. Share any warning information with family, friends, neighbors, and the community.

If you hear an official tsunami warning or detect signs of a tsunami, evacuate at once. A tsunami warning is issued when authorities are certain that a tsunami threat exists, and there may be little time to get out.

You've drilled for this. Grab your tsunami kit and evacuation plan and quickly but calmly move along your escape route. If you have time, take your animals. If it is not safe for you, it is not safe for them. Of course, if you don't have time or cannot carry them or bring them because of extenuating circumstances, do your best to leave them on the highest ground possible and not tied to something or in a cage. Help elderly and needy people along the way, but keep moving.

- Save yourself, not your possessions.
- Grab your tsunami kit.
- Round up your family if they are nearby.
- Follow your planned escape route. Get to higher ground as far inland as possible. Watching a tsunami from the beach or cliffs could put you in grave danger. If you can see the wave, you are too close to escape it.
- Avoid downed power lines and stay away from buildings and bridges from which might fall during an aftershock.
- Stay away until local officials tell you it is safe. A tsunami's series of waves often continue for hours. Do not assume that after one wave the danger is over. The next wave may be larger than the first one.

Let's say you didn't have time to evacuate on time and the tsunami is within sight. Now what? Here are a few scenarios that are your best option depending on where you are and how far away you are from the tsunami.

Go to an upper floor or roof of a building: Do this only if you are trapped and unable to reach higher ground; go to an upper story of a sturdy building or get on its roof.

Climb a tree or pole: The tsunami is on you. Climb up a strong tree. Get as high up as you can. Numerous anecdotes show that people can survive this way but don't make the mistake of getting down without having a clear and safe path to a better escape location because too many times, people get down from trees only to be trapped on the ground by the next wave onslaught.

Climb onto something that floats: This is a lousy escape option because the water will be roily and debris-laden, but it beats trying to swim or float because that's nearly impossible. As you float on your "raft," look for options to jump to something more secure. It's life or death at this point.

More and more coastal communities are building tsunami shelters. These structures are sturdy enough to withstand the force of a tsunami, tall enough to clear the danger zone, and placed in locations where as many people as possible can reach them. See if your area has one and if not, lead the way to get one or more built.

- Most tsunamis are less than ten feet high when they hit land, but they can reach more than one hundred feet high. When a tsunami comes ashore, areas less than twenty-five feet above sea level and within a mile of the sea will be in the greatest danger. However, tsunamis can surge up to ten miles inland.
- The tsunami could resemble a wall of water or a strong flood, but it can have an impressively big wave too. If you

have watched any videos of tsunamis, then you know the incoming wave isn't like a big surfing wave but it can be ten to fifteen feet high, as wide as the harbor, and scary as hell. Listen to the comments of those videoing the impending disaster and you'll hear their incredulity at the power and terror.

• You can also buy survival pods intended to protect you from a tsunami. Survival Capsule is patented as a personal safety system (PSS), designed as a sphere to protect against tsunami events, tornadoes, hurricanes, although they are pricey and have yet to prove their worth. Might be worth checking out.

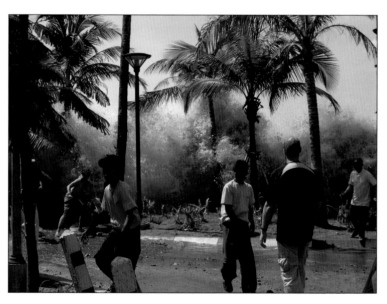

Tsunami waters coming ashore in 2004.

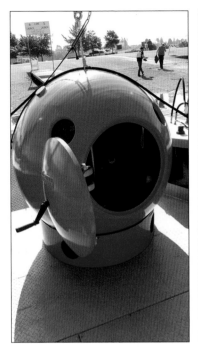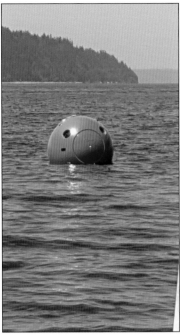

Survival capsule. *Credit: Julian Sharpe, president and CEO of Survival Capsul.*

Aftermath

It's not over until it's over. The first wave came, you survived. Tsunamis come in a series of waves and often, the second and third waves are more powerful than the first. Do not leave a safe haven. Check yourself for injuries and get first aid if necessary before helping injured or trapped persons.

Expect for roads to be wiped out and made unusable by a tsunami. If you're planning on using roads to get where you need to go, think again.

Anticipate aftershocks and additional waves. Earthquakes can have aftershocks for hours and hours, even days. These can cause more tsunamis. And after all, tsunamis come in waves. The waves can last for hours and there could be many waves.

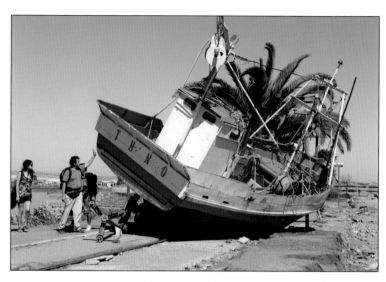

Aftermath of a tsunami in Chile. *Credit: Walter Mooney, US Geological Survey.*

Try to get reliable information. The most important resource in surviving a tsunami is information. If you have phone service, any kind of Internet service to your phone, or a radio, listen to the radio for updates on what is happening. Do not trust word of mouth. It is better to wait than to return too early and be caught by more incoming waves.

Wait for local authorities to issue an "All Clear." Only when you learn that the authorities have provided the "All Clear," should you even consider returning to your home. Remember that roads may be extremely damaged by the tsunami waves and you may have to take alternative routes.

Survival mode doesn't end just because the tsunami has ended. You will encounter panic, debris, destroyed buildings, collapsed bridges, destroyed roads, and broken infrastructure. Unfortunately, you may also encounter injured persons and even dead bodies. Fresh water supplies may be destroyed or disrupted. Ample food supplies will most likely be unavailable. The potential for disease, post-traumatic stress disorder, grief, starvation, and injuries will make the post-tsunami period as dangerous as the tsunami itself. The community emergency plan should have addressed the aftermath and what you'll need to do to protect yourself, your family, and your community. Hopefully, your community plan has provided fresh water, dry shelter, and the means to handle fire hazards such as gas, electricity, and chemicals.

Continue to monitor your NOAA Weather Radio, and stay tuned to a Coast Guard emergency frequency station or a local radio or television station for updated emergency information. The tsunami waves may be over but the earthquake/waves may have damaged roads, bridges, or other places that may be unsafe.

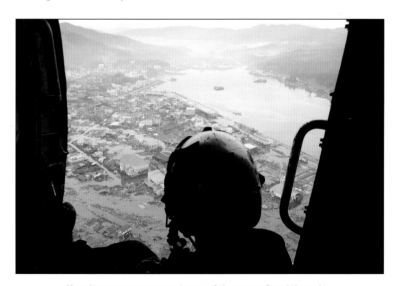

Naval crewman surveys tsunami damage after 9.0 quake.
Credit: Justin Dowd, Naval Air Crewman, 2nd Class.

If you do nothing else:

1. CHECK, CALL, CARE: If people around you are injured, practice CHECK, CALL, CARE. Check the scene to be sure it's safe for you to approach, call for help, and if you are trained, provide first aid to those in need until emergency responders can arrive. Help people who require additional

assistance—infants, elderly people, those without transportation, large families who may need additional help in an
emergency situation, people with disabilities, and others.

2. Let friends and family know you're safe. Register yourself
   as safe on the Safe and Well Website: https://safeandwell.
   communityos.org/cms/index.php

3. If you evacuated, return only when authorities say it is safe
   to do so.

4. Continue listening to local news or a NOAA Weather Radio
   for updated information and instructions.

Caution: Helping others after a flood situation is dangerous. Don't walk
through water that could be deep or is moving rapidly. If someone is
located in a dangerous situation, wait and monitor. Unless someone
is in urgent danger, alert the authorities or community members with
boats or other safety vehicles and monitor the situation. Too many have
lost their lives trying to save others.

Let's be honest: If you saw the aftermath of Hurricane Harvey in
Houston and the surrounding areas, you saw a community, a region,
and a nation come to the rescue of victims. People help people in need.
All the precautions the agencies suggest, all the warnings of things not
to do, well, when people are in need, it's easy to disregard them. Most
people do not risk their own safety to help others because they are
heroes; they do it because we have a human need to do the right thing.
So if you decide to ignore sage advice and become a responder and rescuer, at least be vigilant and somewhat cautious.

Avoid disaster areas. Your presence might hamper rescue and other
emergency operations and put you at further risk from the residual
effects of the tsunami, such as contaminated water, crumbled roads,
landslides, mudflows, and other hazards. Either get safe or help others
to safety. And expect aftershocks. Some aftershocks could be as large as
magnitude 7+ and capable of generating another tsunami. It may take
days, weeks, or months for the aftershocks to subside. If you are with
loved ones, watch how they are acting, how they are handling stress.

If where you are is out of harm's way, stay there. If you are on the
move because of unsafe circumstances, stay out of damaged buildings

and stay out of buildings surrounded by water. The water can be contaminated, or could have reduced the structural stability of the building.

When conditions are all-clear and safe enough to return to your home, don't just rush in. Watch out for fallen power lines or broken gas lines and report them to the utility company immediately. If you smell gas or hear a blowing or hissing noise, don't go in; but if you have entered and hear or smell it, open a window and get everyone outside quickly. Turn off the gas using the outside main valve if you can, and call the gas company from a neighbor's home.

Looting. This is an unfortunate byproduct of any disaster. You are instructed to leave and go to safety but some, a few, will see an opportunity to take advantage of the situation. In the wake of weather disasters, you'll see increased fears about looting, but experts say that while some people do take advantage of the distraction to loot (or commit other crimes), the reality is that it's more in your mind than in your neighborhoods. Houston had fewer than seventy people charged with storm-related crimes and that's out of a population of five million.

So you're back in your house. Check food supplies. Any food that has come in contact with floodwater may be contaminated and should be thrown out. Take pictures for insurance purposes of home damage, both of the buildings and its contents.

To do your cleanup, we recommend wearing long pants, a long-sleeved shirt, and sturdy shoes. The most common injury following a disaster, especially a flood, is cut feet. We recommend quick-dry shirts and pants; our go-tos are generic quick-dry fishing shirts and fishing pants.

Use battery-powered lanterns or flashlights when examining buildings. Battery-powered lighting is the safest and easiest to use, and it does not present a fire hazard for the user, occupants, or building. DO NOT USE CANDLES. Do not turn on the electricity first. Examine the house before you do any that could result in injury.

Examine walls, floors, doors, staircases, and windows to make sure that the building is not in danger of collapsing. If you have any doubts, do not remain. Inspect foundations for cracks or other damage. Cracks and damage to a foundation can render a building uninhabitable.

Fire is the most common hazard after a tsunami flood, so look for fire hazards. There may be leaking gas lines, flooded electrical circuits, submerged furnaces, or electrical appliances. You might encounter flammable or explosive materials. If you smell gas, if you hear a blowing or hissing noise, open a window and get everyone outside quickly. If you can, turn off the gas yourself at the main outside valve. If you don't know where it is, call the gas company and keep everyone away from the house (and warn your neighbors, too.) Do not light up a cigarette.

Look for electrical system damage. If you see sparks or broken or frayed wires, or if you smell burning insulation, turn off the electricity at the main fuse box or circuit breaker. If you have to step in water to get to the fuse box or circuit breaker, call an electrician first for advice. Electrical equipment should be checked and dried before being returned to service.

If you have water still standing in your house, and the electricity is on, you could put yourself or family in danger. Don't risk electrocution. Call an electrician and plumber.

Animals may have come into the house or building looking to get away from the flood. They could be pets, or they could be wild animals. Either way, keep an eye out. Look for poisonous snakes especially. Before you just start picking up this and that to throw away, use a stick to poke through debris. FYI: Hurricane Harvey's floods found wild creatures in houses, including a nine-foot alligator. Surprise!

Take photos (and have another person take some too, just in case.) Redundancy doesn't hurt. Get multiple angles of any damage to property and contents. You'll need these for insurance purposes.

- Open doors and windows so the place can dry out. If you have electricity and no standing water, use fans to aid drying.
- With all the water, you may have loose plaster, drywall, and ceilings that could fall.
- Find a shovel. Shovel that mud before it becomes concrete-like. You may not be able to take the debris and mud to a

disposal station, so find a corner of your house far enough away that you don't attract mice or insects; far enough away that the smell doesn't get into the house.

- Some recommend that if water has been in your house for any length of time, you rip out the sheet rock right away to avoid mold buildup.
- Don't trust any food that could have been exposed to any floodwater. It might be contaminated. Throw it away.

Tsunami Myths

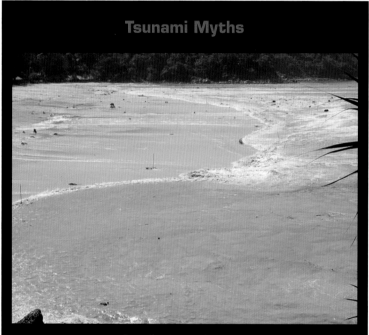

Receding tsunami waters.

Myth: A tsunami is a single wave. Once it has occurred you are safe.

This is false. A tsunami is a series of waves. There may be five to twenty waves that come during fixed periods which are typically ten minutes to twenty hours. The first waves are typically small, and subsequent waves become larger. Therefore, if you don't get washed away by the first wave, you still need to stay away from the shoreline to escape the others.

Myth: There's not much that you can do to avoid a tsunami.

This is also false. If you happen to be on the seashore and the tide suddenly goes out and you see fish flopping in the mud and sand, this typically means that a tsunami is coming. You should move to higher ground immediately. Fish are smart creatures and they never flop around when low tides happen daily. The water will often recede as much as one thousand yards from the beach before the first tsunami wave hits. However, there is no guarantee that this will always happen either.

Myth: A tsunami looks like a big television-show style surfing wave.

False. What makes a tsunami so destructive is not the height of the wave, but the large volume of water that pours out onto the beach. The distinguishing characteristic of a tsunami is that it is a long period wave—very broad but not necessarily particularly high, even at the seashore.

Myth: Tsunamis only occur in the Pacific Ocean.

False. As most people now know, a tsunami can occur in any ocean. Luckily, tsunamis find it more difficult to propagate in the Atlantic Ocean because of its shallower depth and the Mid-Atlantic Ridge. However, because of its smaller size, any tsunami in the Atlantic will also have less distance to travel. The strength of a wave is roughly inversely proportional to the distance from the source. So any tsunami in the Atlantic will be more localized, but you may get little warning.

Myth: If you can grab onto a solid object, you are likely to survive a tsunami.

False. Okay, there are the few anecdotes of survivors who held on to something and lived but they are the exception to the rule. You may not drown or even get washed away if you are holding on to something solid, but you may well be struck by pieces of wood, branches, rocks, vehicles, and other objects traveling in the water at 30 miles per hour. One cubic yard of sea water weighs 1,727 pounds. A tsunami wave moving at 30 miles per hour has kinetic energy equivalent to a Ford pickup truck traveling at 20 miles per hour. Normal humans can't hold on when confronted with this kind of energy. Holding on to an object will be even more difficult if the water is cold.

Myth: Volcanoes and underwater landslides can produce tsunamis.

This is true. Tsunamis are caused by sudden, large-scale vertical displacement of water. Displacement can be by earthquake (in 87 percent of cases) but also by landslide, avalanche, volcano, and even meteorite.

Myth: You can surf a tsunami.

False. You cannot surf a tsunami. The wave is just too broad, and not high enough with not enough energy.

Myth: Tsunamis are giant walls of water.

Partly true. Occasionally, tsunamis can form walls of water (known as tsunami bores) but tsunamis normally have the appearance of a fast-rising and fast-receding flood. They can be similar to a tide cycle occurring in just ten to sixty minutes instead of twelve hours.

Myth: Boats should move to the protection of a bay or harbor during a tsunami.

False. Bays and harbors will not provide protection during a tsunami. The powerful waves usually pummel anything and everything in a bay/harbor.

Myth: A tsunami is the same thing as a tidal wave.

False. Tidal waves are regular ocean waves, and are caused by the tides. These waves are caused by the interaction of the pull of the moon's gravity on the earth. A "tidal wave" is a term used in common folklore to mean the same thing as a tsunami, but is not the same thing.

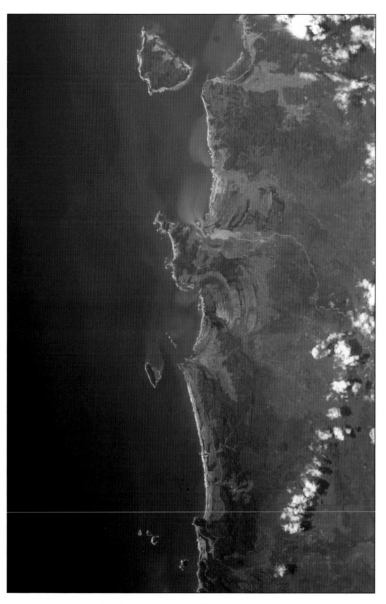

Aerial view of damage in Sumatra, Indonesia.
Credit: Expedition 10 crew member on International Space Station.

Tsunami Facts

1. A tsunami is a series of ocean waves caused by an underwater earthquake, landslide, or volcanic eruption. More rarely, a tsunami can be generated by a giant meteor impact with the ocean. These waves can reach heights of over one hundred feet.

2. The first wave of a tsunami is usually not the strongest; successive waves get bigger and stronger.

3. Tsunamis can travel at speeds of about 500 miles or 805 kilometers an hour, almost as fast as a jet plane.

4. Scientists can accurately estimate the time when a tsunami will arrive almost anywhere around the world based on calculations using the depth of the water, distances from one place to another, and the time that the earthquake or other event occurred.

5. One cubic yard of sea water weighs about 1,700 pounds. That is nearly one ton. A tsunami wave moving at 30 miles per hour has kinetic energy equivalent to the solid mass of medium sized SUV traveling at 20 miles per hour.

6. The highest tidal waves are found in the Bay of Fundy, in the Canadian province of New Brunswick, where the water level can rise with the tide by fifty feet.

7. A tsunami wave isn't too much different in height compared to other waves in the ocean (about one meter only out from the shore). But it is quite long so it piles up when approaches land. That is why a tsunami generally goes unnoticed in the open ocean. In addition, tsunamis move the depth of the ocean and not just its surface. That is why tsunamis contain such powerful energy and move at great speed for unbelievable distances, still remaining powerful enough to cause a devastating damage along coastlines. Tsunamis can also travel up rivers and streams that lead to the ocean.

8. Most tsunami waves are less than ten feet tall.

9. Twenty-four tsunamis have caused damage in the United States and its territories in the past two hundred years.

10. Since 1946, six tsunamis in the United States have killed more than 350 people and caused significant property damage in Hawaii, Alaska, and along the West Coast. Tsunamis have also occurred in Puerto Rico and the Virgin Islands.

11. The most devastating effect of tsunamis is that after one wave hits and causes damage, the water recedes as the next wave approaches, taking with it the debris associated with the first wave. Then, when the next wave hits all the water and debris moves inland yet again with even more force and weight behind it causing even more damage and devastation.

12. Tsunamis aren't restricted to oceans—they can also occur in large lakes.

13. The highest tsunami wave ever recorded was over 1,700 feet tall in Lituya Bay, Alaska, caused by a landslide in 1958.

Helpful Resources for Tsunami Preparation

You can get advance warning. Should an official tsunami alert be issued, you will be notified via e-mail and/or a text message if you subscribe to a service. Some are free, while others charge a fee. Here are a few we found.

Tsunami-Alarm-System.com
SMS (short message service) alert sent to mobile phone; $40 per year.

Tsunami-Warn.com
SMS alert sent to mobile phone; $29 per month.

CWarn.org
SMS alert sent to mobile phone; free.

ioc3.unesco.org/itic/contents.php?id=142
Sends alert via e-mail; free.

sslearthquake.usgs.gov/ens
Sends earthquake (not tsunami) notifications via e-mail and SMS text messages; free.

ptwc.weather.gov
Website you can access 24/7 for real-time status of any tsunami alerts. It does not send you an alert, but you can get data immediately and monitor alerts.

CHAPTER FIVE

AVALANCHES

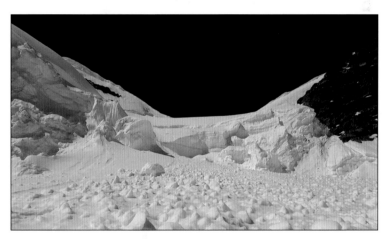

Credit: Simon Steinberger.

If you've ever watched a video of an avalanche, then you know they are capricious, sudden, and powerful forces, moving with breathtaking speed down steep mountains and destroying large swaths of forest. Between 1975 and 2000 almost seventeen thousand people have been killed in landslides (rock and dirt) and avalanches (snow and rock and dirt) worldwide. Avalanches kill more than 150 people worldwide each year and over twenty-five deaths annually in America. In 90 percent of avalanche accidents, the victim or someone in the victim's party causes the snow slide. Asphyxiation is the most common cause of death in an avalanche, claiming about 90 percent of victims. Because, only a few seconds after an avalanche the snow quickly turns into ice, freezing hard as cement. Eighty-nine percent of victims are men.

We have pretty good statistics for deaths and injuries in avalanches, but have you wondered how many escape an avalanche by the skin of their teeth? It's a loose calculation but experts believe that for every death, about ten people are caught in an avalanche of snow and ice and somehow escape with their lives.

If you get buried in an avalanche, you only have a 27 percent chance of survival after thirty-five minutes. After one hour, only one in three victims buried in an avalanche is found alive. Statistics show that 93 percent of avalanche victims survive if dug out within fifteen minutes. Suffocation is responsible for most avalanche deaths, and trauma is the cause of 24 percent of the deaths. The last one percent are killed by hypothermia. Avalanche victims are typically backcountry recreationalists: skiers, snowboarders, climbers, and snowmobilers. With the rising popularity of snowmobiling, snowmobilers now account for twice as many avalanche fatalities as other groups. Since snowmobilers weigh more, the risk of stressing the weak layer in a snowpack and setting off an avalanche is greater.

Avalanches are caused by four factors: a steep slope, snow cover, a weak layer in the snow cover, and a trigger. By the way, it's a myth that noise triggers avalanches. Avalanches can be triggered by wind, rain, warming temperatures, snow, and earthquakes. They can also be triggered by skiers, snowmobiles, hikers, vibrations from machinery or construction. We mostly think of avalanches and skiers or snowboarders but if you are staying in a hotel or home near a snowy mountain, well, you could be in danger too. Avalanches are most common in mountainous areas of Utah, Alaska, Idaho, Montana, Alaska, California, Washington, and Oregon.

Steeper slopes carry a greater risk of a snowslide. Slab avalanches are the most dangerous type of avalanche and account for as much as 90 percent of all avalanche-related fatalities. Slab avalanches are formed when snow gets deposited by wind. When they fracture, they look like a heavy block of snow cut out from the side of the mountain and can vary in thickness from a few inches to a few feet. A slab avalanche is essentially an entire cohesive plate of snow that breaks free and slides across a weaker layer and can accelerate to between 60 miles per hour and 80 miles per hour in as little as five seconds. The heavy dry slab avalanches can top 100 to 200 miles per hour at top speed but the wet snow avalanches move much slower, perhaps in the 20 miles per hour range.

The other types of avalanche are loose snow avalanches which are common in steep terrains and usually occur in fresh-fallen snow; powder snow avalanches which form a cloud of powder over the avalanche; and wet snow avalanches which tend to move slowly (heavy with water) but can still be destructive of trees, rocks, and property.

Even though we cause most of the avalanches that affect us, these forces of nature do occur naturally as well. They might happen when there is an increased load of snowfall. They might happen from the melting from solar radiation, or it might be from rain, rock, or ice falling, or even earthquakes.

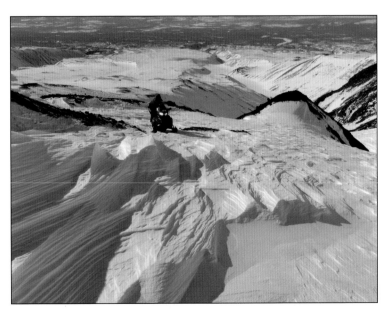

Snowmobiling, a major factor in triggering avalanches. *Credit: Pixabay.*

Trigger points that activate an avalanche are usually at locations where the top slab of snow is thinner. Most avalanches occur on slopes with angles between 30 and 45 degrees (38 degrees is the most common slope for an avalanche.) Steeper slopes tend to slough snow when it gets too deep so that a snowpack doesn't build up.

Avalanche risk is at its greatest twenty-four hours following a snowfall and this is because often, fresh snowfall does not bond well to the underlying snow. This new snow on old snow is the recipe for a slab avalanche. If you get a foot or greater of fresh snow you have a much greater avalanche risk than snowfall cover less than a foot deep.

A great resource for avalanche information, maps, and up-to-date avalanche warnings and dangers is www.avalanche.org.

Preparation

Avalanche Survival tends to fall into five categories: Education, Equipment, Observation, Traveling in Numbers, and Survival Techniques.

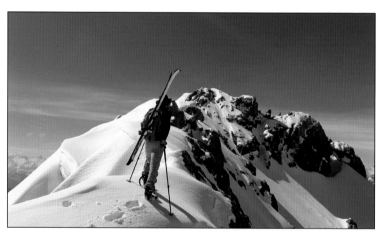

Be avalanche aware when skiing in the backcountry. *Credit: Pixabay.*

1. Education

If you are planning to travel in backcountry, it makes sense to take an avalanche safety course. Route-finding, avalanche safety, and rescue skills are the basics you will need to know. If you are in mountainous country, you'll find many organizations that will provide intensive training courses for snowmobilers, skiers, and snowboarders on how to spot avalanche risk, avoid avalanches, survive if caught in one, and how to rescue each other.

Instructors can show you how factors like precipitation, wind, temperature, snow stability, and terrain set up possible avalanches. You will learn to recognize how slope steepness, orientation, and underlying rock affect conditions. They teach you to check snowpack stability, route recognition, and how to dig pits. Safety classes also teach you how to use beacons, probes, and shovels (yes, there are efficiency techniques and group strategies). Get to know the danger rating definitions for the five international avalanche danger levels: 1 (low), 2 (moderate), 3 (considerable), 4 (high), 5 (extreme).

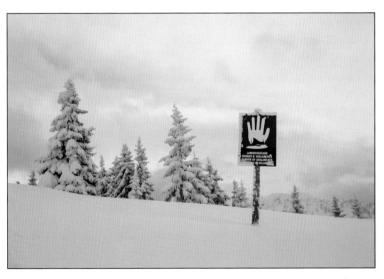

Avoid avalanche danger areas and observe warning signs. *Credit: Pixabay.*

Before you head out on the slope, you have several things you need to do:

Read the official avalanche forecast bulletin for your area. Travel with people who have a similar approach, education, observation, and sense of safety. Have all the right equipment at hand. Don't get out there and remember you left something at home. You might have to save a life today (and it might be yours).

Have you trained with your safety equipment? If you don't know how to use it, you're taking a big chance. Go out with a friend beforehand and get familiar with your gear. Doesn't hurt to refresh yourself every so often either. Have your phone with you? Does it have the phone numbers of local rescue services and other important contacts? Is it fully charged? Is it in a dry pocket or in a waterproof case? Do you and your friends have a good idea of the area and routes you'll be traversing? Are one of you carrying maps or a guidebook or a GPS mapping device with you? Do you feel comfortable on how to identify slopes of 30 degrees or more? And make sure to talk to local professionals to get every bit of local information on your area and any risk involved.

The factors that increase (or diminish) the likelihood of an avalanche occurring are surprisingly complex—things like weather, sun, temperature, wind, the angle of the mountain's slope, and snowpack conditions. The avalanche hazard level can fluctuate daily and even hourly as conditions change. This means that the ability to scout for potential avalanches takes a good amount of both education and preparation.

2. Equipment

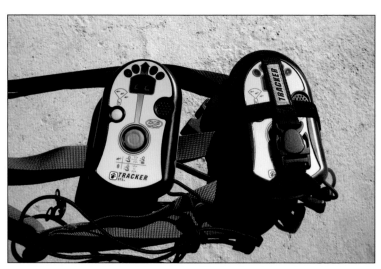

An avalanche transceiver helps rescuers locate a person buried by snow.
Credit: Bodhisattwa, creativecommons.org_licenses_by-sa_4.0, Wikimedia Commons.

The most basic equipment each backcountry traveler should carry include helmet, receiver (you'll see it called a transceiver) and probe, and shovel. Your helmet should have a face shield and it makes sense to have a good seal around the neck. To carry the other gear, you need a backpack for skiing or if you snowmobile, have your bag easily accessible for all your gear. You want your receiver on your person of course. The case can be made that no matter if you are skiing, snowboarding, or snowmobiling, you should carry all your gear on your person in case your snowmobile is buried or out of range.

Avalanche Transceiver (Beacon)

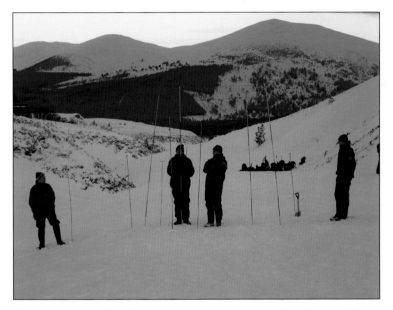

A probe and shovel used by a rescue teams during search-and-rescue drills. Credit: Iain Lees, creativecommons.org_licenses_by-sa_2.0, Wikimedia Commons.

This should always be on your person in avalanche terrain. These devices send snow-penetrating radio waves on a standard frequency all the time. If someone is caught in an avalanche, switch yours to receive to hone-in on your partner's position. Easier to use than ever, these devices still require proper technique and practice. Beacons transmit a radio frequency to a receiver or another beacon. This enables your rescuers to pinpoint exactly where you are underneath the snow before they start digging. Some jackets or clothing have embedded technology that can help rescuers to locate a buried skier.

Probe

Locate where your partner is buried by the avalanche. A probe will help you dig in the right spot so you're not digging wastefully. Every second counts. A probe is also great for tracking snow depth and locating crevasses.

Shovel

Dig hard, dig efficiently! Digging in the packed snow is going to be difficult, so make sure you have the right kind of shovel and know the proper technique. Besides, what if you got caught out overnight? With your shovel you can check out snow depth or dig a snow shelter and survive. Most avalanche-shovels fit on your back.

Avalanche airbag (balloon system)

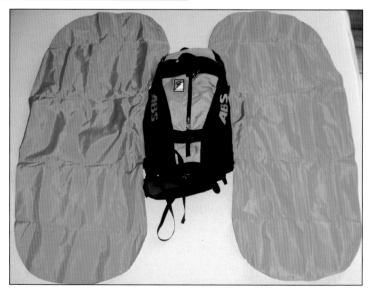

An avalanche airbag. *Credit: Nolispanmo, creativecommons.org_licenses_ by-sa_3.0, Wikimedia Commons.*

An ABS (airbag system) is an attempt to thwart getting buried by an avalanche. You wear the airbag and if you are in avalanche danger, you immediately activate the bag. It blows up like a balloon and while it might not keep you from getting buried, the idea is that it keeps you closer to the surface. Experts say the results are mixed and the costs are still high enough to be prohibitive. If you can afford it, buy and use the ABS.

Dress warmly, knowing that if you or a buddy get caught in an avalanche, it could be hours (or longer) before you can get to a warm place again. Pack a small first aid kit too, if you can. Skiers should wear releasable bindings and not use the pole straps. Snowboarders should rig their bindings with a ripcord to release the snowboard in a hurry.

Another tool that is showing promise in avalanche survival is the AvaLung, a snorkel-type device that aids breathing if you are buried. The AvaLung uses a mouthpiece to draw oxygen and dispel carbon dioxide. Since asphyxiation is the major killer when buried, any time you can buy gives you a great chance at surviving until you can be rescued.

3. Observation

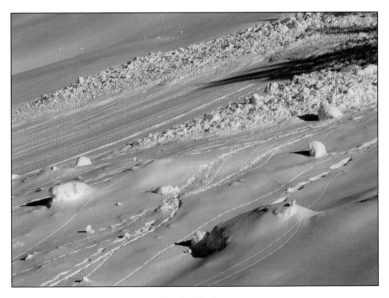

Credit: Pixabay.

The most important element of avalanche safety is to use your education to observe the signs of an impending or possible avalanche so you can avoid one altogether. When you combine all your education and observational skills in a group effort, you maximize your chances of enjoying the backcountry with no avalanche event. Check your local forecast the night before and morning of your possible trek. Study where the most dangerous slopes might be. Make sure everyone in the group is on the same page.

Call or get online to check the area avalanche report. The many mountainous areas in North America typically have avalanche centers that issue regular avalanche advisories. This gives you an easy, overall view of snow stability for your area. There are some smartphone apps that display updated information.

The best indicator of possible avalanches are other avalanches. You can't get much more obvious than that. But it's surprising how often

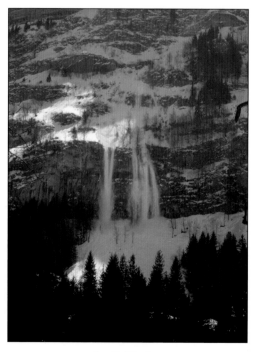

Credit: Pixabay.

people miss this clue. Another good indicator of worsening avalanche conditions include any weather change that is rapid, such as recent rapid loading of new or windblown snow, recent rapid warming, recent rapid melting, and rain on new snow.

When driving, observe any warning signs advising about avalanches. Drive carefully in avalanche areas. Avalanches may hit or cover the road without warning. Head on a swivel. Obey road closures. If an avalanche blocks the highway, remain in your vehicle with seat belts on and call emergency services and wait for assistance. It is easier to find a car in the snow than it is to find a person. If you can reverse safely, do so but make sure to alert other drivers and call emergency services.

On the initial part of your party going into the backcountry, especially if it is an ascent, be observant. Traverse low-angle ridges, near dense forest, away from dangerous slopes when possible. Move from safe zone to safe zone, and if you must cross areas that seem avalanche-prone, spread out so not everyone is exposed to danger.

Listen for collapsing snow. When you hear the snowpack collapse, your ear just told you that things are unstable. Stay off of steep slopes. Don't go underneath steep slopes. Listen for cracking or whooping snow. Recent wind loading is the culprit for cracking snow and in fact, the longer the crack, the more dangerous it is.

When it's time to let her rip, have fun in the backcountry, but don't become un-observant. Keep using the same evaluation skills you have been, keep identifying safe zones versus danger zones and maintain safety for the entire party. Don't be afraid to stop and judge snow stability, to back off a line or an area, and don't get careless on that "last run" of the day.

4. Traveling in Numbers

When traveling in backcountry, always travel in a group. It's a good idea to have an experienced group leader. Always stay within view of your group.

Is everyone geared up? Knowledgeable about your routes? Watching carefully for any possible dangers? As each person is about

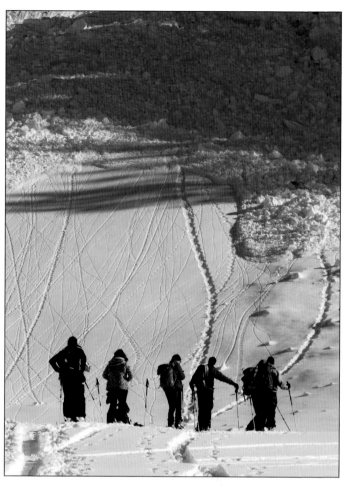

Travel in numbers when in the backcountry. *Credit: Pixabay.*

to commence their fun route, have you talked it over with the group to minimize any triggering? Before you commit to your route, visualize what an avalanche would look like on the slope. Talk about it with your group. Where can you move to reduce your avalanche hazard? Your party should have an evacuation plan of sorts and be equipped for winter travel with warm clothes, snacks, and first aid in case things go awry. There is strength in numbers especially in an avalanche, even more so in avalanche rescue.

5. Survival Techniques

See below.

Survival

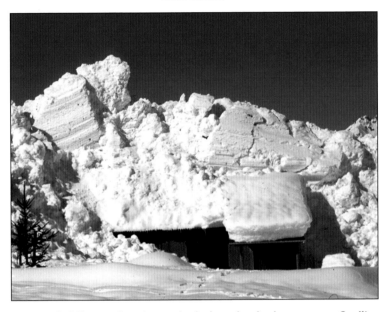

Homes, buildings, and roads can also be in avalanche danger zones. *Credit: Scientif38, creativecommons.org_licenses_by-sa_3.0, Wikimedia Commons.*

If you're caught in an avalanche, the best thing you can do is try to get out of the avalanche! Sounds good, right? But how do you do that?

First, what happens when you are caught in an avalanche? You are wearing a helmet because once it starts, you might be tossed around, career roughly into a tree, or get hit by debris. This maelstrom will occur suddenly and survivors say the sensation is like being caught in a high-speed washing machine. If you can, jump uphill, above the fracture. If you can't do that, run or slide to the side of the avalanche. We know, easier said than done, but if you can, do it. If you're on skis or a snowboard, head downhill first to gather some speed, and then veer to the side and off the slab. If you're on a snowmobile, keep going in the direction you were going and throttle it to get off the sliding snow. The presiding idea is to get off the slab, out of the avalanche, do whatever you can to escape.

If none of that works and you are in the tumult of the avalanche, drop your ski poles or abandon your snowmobile—you don't want to have those things weighing you down, twisting in the snowslide and hurting you, or in the case of the snowmobile, landing on top of you. You do not want your skis on as you tumble nor do you want your ski poles attached to your wrists. You need to be light and buoyant. Here's the tough part: you need to free yourself up while deploying your ABS and finding your AvaLung. And that's not all . . . you should be trying a few survival techniques.

Swim. Swim with all your might and ferocity. Try to stay on top. Experts will tell you to lay back and do the backstroke to avoid the toe (tip) of the avalanche, the most turbulent part of any avalanche. But do whatever it takes to avoid being buried. You may be disoriented in the initial thrust but as it slows, fight to get to the top. Avalanche debris has a similar mass to setting concrete, and further movement becomes impossible.

Dig. Some survivors suggest digging in with your feet to slow your descent. Some have also said that rolling their body like a log helped them get to the side of the flow.

Reach. Try to keep one arm above your head, above your body on your violent descent. This is easier said than done, but try to keep one arm above your head as the avalanche tosses you around. If you can pull this off, it will be easier for rescuers to spot you if your arm or hand is sticking up out of the snow; and if your arm is out of the snow, you'll know which direction is up.

If you're wearing an ABS backpack, pull the trigger and release your airbag. Hopefully this will keep you on the surface. Never wear wrist loops in a potential avalanche zone.

Try to keep your nose and mouth free from snow and use your arms to establish space around your face before it finally stops. Push machinery, equipment, or heavy objects away from you to avoid injury.

When a slide stops it will quickly settle like concrete, so as the snow begins to set up, take a big breath. This expands your chest, which can give you a little extra breathing room as the snow hardens around you. If rescuers can dig out the victim within fifteen minutes, there is a 90 percent chance of survival, so time is of the essence. After that the odds drop quickly. Only 20 percent of buried victims are still alive after forty-five minutes, and beyond two hours, few ever survive. Everything you can do to aid the rescuers helps your chances at survival.

As the avalanche slows to a stop, push yourself towards the surface. Attempt to make an air pocket in front of your face using one arm and if you are able, push your other arm towards the surface.

Once the Avalanche Has Buried You

If the avalanche buries you, you survived any serious trauma, and you're still alive, well, you are lucky. About 33 percent of avalanche victims are killed by trauma. But your window for survival is small so hopefully, you've done all the preparation and education, including wearing a receiver. If you are able, try to create an air pocket by putting your arm across your face as the mass slows. Every little bit of breathing room is vital so this doesn't become your snowy tomb.

Because you are buried, trapped from a tumultuous event, you probably won't know which way is up. You'll also be in panic mode—who wouldn't be? The snow may be so packed you cannot move your fingers or expand your chest to take a big breath. But the calmer you are, the slower you will breathe and the less quickly you'll use up the oxygen. You will want to turn your head side to side and create whatever little air pockets you can so you can breathe.

Don't yell either. It'll waste energy and oxygen and since snow is insulating, rescuers are not likely to hear you. If you've worn your beacon, rescuers will be on the way, and you'll get pulled out of the debris soon. If you hear a rescuer nearby, a quick loud shout is worth the risk.

Rely on Your Buddies

Observation is the key. If you see the avalanche occur and your buddy get caught in it, watch closely to see if you can follow your buddy's path

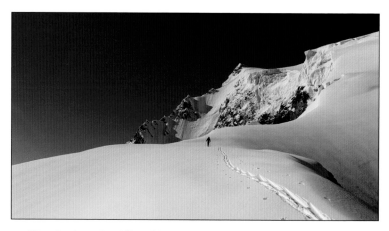

When backcountry skiing with others, traverse the mountain one at a time.
Credit: Simon Steinberger.

and where he or she has stopped. This is where practice with your avalanche rescue gear, education from experts, and team coordination all coalesce.

Aftermath

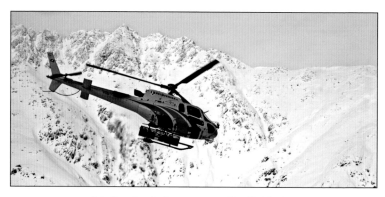

A helicopter during a rescue. *Credit: Pixabay.*

You've just witnessed one or more of your party get caught up in an avalanche? First, stay calm. Second, keep your eyes on them. Watch your buddy carefully from the time they are swept away until they aren't visible beneath the snow. Keep particular care to note where they were swept away to where they disappeared until the avalanche comes to a stop. Knowing this area will give you an idea of where they might have ended up. After the avalanche has come to a full stop, go and find them. You are trained in using your avalanche beacon and metal probe so you can hone in on where they are buried. Waste no time. Start digging.

Because asphyxiation is the most common underlying cause of avalanche deaths, the more quickly a victim can be located and dug out, the higher the chance of survival. Your first instinct might be to go for help. Do not go for help. You and your buddies are the best hope. We cannot emphasize enough that time is of the essence.

Let's just say your buddy was in a hurry, and careless, and forgot to wear a beacon. This is one reason that the continued sightline of their path is important. Look for clues on the surface. Can you find their skis, hat, gloves, or ski poles? Many times, these provide a line to where the victim is buried. Because of the dynamics of moving snow, victims often get buried in certain places—above rocks and trees, on the outside of the avalanche path if it curves. If you lost track of your buddy, probe these spots.

So your buddy wore a beacon and you have located it under the snow? Digging takes a while because you may have to move a lot of snow and it's usually hard packed. If you can determine that the victim is buried just under two to three feet of snow, start digging furiously to reach them. But if they're buried in snow that's deeper than that, you should employ different digging strategies, depending on how many people you have with you.

If you have several available diggers, form a "V." The front person does the digging, and moves the displaced snow just a little ways behind him or her. The two people behind the digger then push the snow to the people behind them, and on down the line. The front person is rotated every minute or so, so that the digger remains fresh. If it's just you and the buried victim, you'll want to employ the "strategic digging" method. When you locate someone with a probe and know exactly where they are in the snow, you don't want to dig straight down into where the probe is sticking out of the snow. The probe might be at their legs, and when you dig down, you may shovel snow behind you and onto their air pocket, collapsing it. Then you'll end up with a cone-shaped hole that's not at their airway.

Instead, shift your position to downhill from the probe, about one to two times the length of the depth in which the victim is buried. Start digging into the side of the slope, straight into where you think your victim is buried. To save more time and energy, shovel the snow out to the side instead of behind you, until the snow rises to your waist—then start moving it downhill. Uncover their face and clear an airway as soon as you can.

Once you locate the victim, before you pull them out, clear their airway and make sure they can breathe properly. Remove them from the snowpack and lay them down where you can continue to clear their airway, perform CPR, and administer first aid.

CHAPTER SIX

BLIZZARDS AND OTHER WINTER-RELATED STORMS

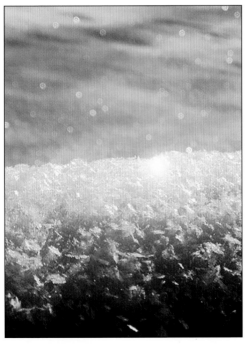

Snowflakes. *Credit: Florian.b, Wikimedia Commons.*

Some veterans of big storms will laugh at those of us who line up in stores for supplies and groceries at the sign of the first little snowflake. But if we are about to endure a blizzard, ice storm, big snowstorm, or any storm that is not your garden-variety winter occurrence, then we feel justified for all that time spent in line at the grocery store. For all those other times when nary a snowflake fell, well, we plead guilty.

Big winter storms can shut down vast regions and entire cities. They can paralyze emergency response, cripple public transportation, halt utilities like power and water, cause travel closures making roads impassable, and cause whiteouts where you and you alone are responsible for you and your family's safety until everything comes back online. Cold temperatures, power outages, wind, wind chill, exposure that can bring about frostbite or hypothermia, other injuries, and other deaths may occur from exposure, dangerous road conditions, and carbon monoxide poisoning and other conditions. The Great Plains of the United States tends to be the region that experiences blizzards most often, but if an area anywhere in America gets snow, a blizzard, ice storm, or big snowstorm are possibilities.

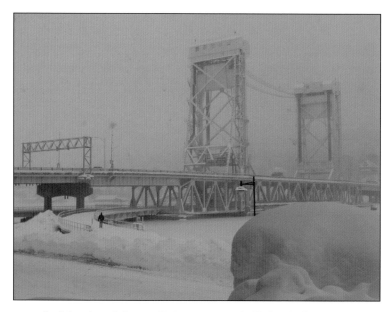

A winter storm brings a city to a near standstill. *Credit: Chris Light, creativecommons.org licenses by-sa 4.0, Wikimedia Commons.*

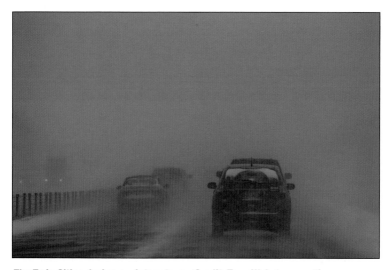

The Twin Cities during a winter storm. *Credit: Tony Webster, creativecommons. org licenses by 2.0 ,Wikimedia Commons.*

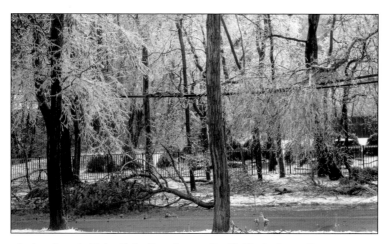

An ice storm in Tinton Falls, New Jersey. *Credit: Shortynj, creativecommons. org licenses by 2.5, Wikimedia Commons.*

The extreme conditions of blizzard and ice storm are born from winter storms. A winter storm occurs when there is significant precipitation and the temperature is low enough that precipitation forms as sleet or snow, or when rain turns to ice. A winter storm can range from freezing rain and ice, to moderate snowfall over a few hours, to heavy snowfall over a few days, or to a raging blizzard that lasts for several days. Many of these winter storms have dangerously low temperatures.

Blizzards can create life-threatening conditions. Traveling by automobile can become difficult or even impossible due to "whiteout" conditions and drifting snow. Whiteout conditions occur most often with major storms that produce a drier, more powdery snow. In this situation, it doesn't even need to be snowing to produce whiteout conditions, as the snow which is already on the ground is blown around, reducing the visibility to nearly zero at times.

An ice storm can quickly paralyze a region and is so dangerous that merely walking out of your door is a huge risk to your survival. During an ice storm, power often goes out. Power lines and tree branches simply cannot take the weight of ice build-up so they come crashing down. And when power goes out during an ice storm, repair crews can't make the necessary repairs until after the storm has passed—which could take a long time.

Bear in mind that it is a really dangerous thing to have no power during an ice storm. During a snowstorm, it is still possible to travel from one place to another; however, your ability to move to a much safer place is dramatically decreased during an ice storm, when road conditions are a lot riskier. Therefore, be sure you have means to keep warm during an ice storm and there's no power. Consider also that the pipes in your home may freeze.

The strong winds and cold temperatures accompanying blizzards can combine to create another danger. The wind chill factor is the amount of cooling one "feels" due to the combination of wind and temperature. During blizzards, with the combination of cold temperatures and strong winds, very low wind chill values can occur. It is not uncommon in the Midwest to have wind chills below -60 degrees Fahrenheit during blizzard conditions. Exposure to such low wind chill values can result in frostbite or hypothermia. For more information, go to the NWS wind chill web page, http://www.nws.noaa.gov/om/cold/wind_chill.shtml.

People should never venture out in blizzards, nor should they continue to travel if a storm is upgraded to a blizzard. To protect yourself

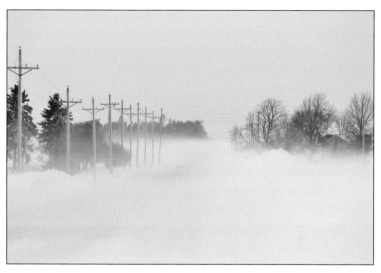

Blizzard conditions.
Credit: FLKR by TOM, creativecommons.org. licenses.by.2.0.

from the effects of winter storms, including blizzards, the National Weather Service suggests the following:

While heavy snowfalls and severe cold often accompany blizzards, they are not required to create a blizzard condition. Sometimes strong winds pick up snow that has already fallen, generating a ground blizzard. Officially, the National Weather Service defines a blizzard as a storm which contains large amounts of falling or blowing snow, with winds in excess of 35 miles per hour and visibilities of less than a quarter mile for an extended period of time (at least three hours). When these conditions are expected, the National Weather Service will issue a "Blizzard Warning." When these conditions are not expected to occur simultaneously, but one or two of these conditions are expected, a "Winter Storm Warning" or "Heavy Snow Warning" may be issued.

Blizzard conditions often develop on the northwest side of an intense storm system. The difference between the lower pressure in the storm and the higher pressure to the west creates a tight pressure gradient, meaning the difference in pressure between two locations, which in turn results in very strong winds. These strong winds pick up available snow from the ground, or blow any snow which is falling, creating very low visibilities and the potential for significant drifting of snow.

Stuck Between High and Low Pressure

Blizzard winds are created when a strong low pressure area is close to a strong high pressure area. The air "tries" to flow from high pressure to low pressure, but the turning of the Earth causes the air to turn to the right (in the Northern Hemisphere), and the wind ends up flowing around the low pressure area, rather than directly toward it.

The difference between the lower pressure in the storm and the higher pressure to the west creates a tight pressure gradient, or difference in pressure between two locations, which in turn results in strong winds. The strong winds blow falling snow and pick snow up from the ground, which cut visibility and create big snow drifts.

Each year, hundreds of Americans are injured or killed by exposure to cold, vehicle accidents on wintry roads, and fires caused by the improper use of heaters. Learn what to do to keep your loved ones safe during blizzards and other winter storms.

Types of NWS Designations

Watch: Issued when conditions are favorable for hazardous winter weather or non-precipitation hazard to develop but its occurrence, location, and/or timing are still uncertain.

Warning: Issued when hazardous winter weather or non-precipitation event is occurring, is imminent, or has a high probability of occurrence. A warning is used for conditions posing a threat to life or property.

Advisory: Issued for less serious conditions that are occurring, imminent, or have a high probability of occurrence, that can cause significant inconvenience and, if caution is not exercised, could lead to situations that threaten life or property.

Blizzard Warning: Sustained winds or frequent gusts of 35 miles per hour or more, and visibility frequently below a quarter mile in considerable snow and/or blowing snow, and above conditions are expected to prevail for three hours or longer.

Winter Storm Warning: Issued when more than one winter hazard is involved producing life threatening conditions, such as a combination of heavy snow, strong winds producing widespread blowing and drifting snow, freezing rain, or wind chill.

Heavy Snow Warning Criteria:

Above 8,500 feet	12 inches/12 hours	18 inches/24 hours
7,000 to 8,500 feet	8 inches/12 hours*	12 inches/24 hours*
5,000 to 7,000 feet	6 inches/12 hours	10 inches/24 hours
Below 5,000 feet	2 inches/12 hours	4 inches/24 hours

Snow Advisory Criteria:

Above 8,500 feet	6 to 12 inches/12 hours	12 to 18 inches/24 hours
7,000 to 8,500 feet	4 to 8 inches/12 hours*	8 to 12 inches/24 hours*
5,000 to 7,000 feet	3 to 6 inches/12 hours	6 to 10 inches/24 hours
Below 5,000 feet	1 to 2 inches/12 hours	2 inches/24 hours*

*or snow accumulation in any location where it is a rare event.

Blowing Snow Advisory Criteria: Visibility frequently at or below a quarter mile.

High Wind Warning Criteria: Issued for strong winds not associated with severe local storms. These include: gradient, mesoscale, and channeled winds; Foehn/Chinook/downslope winds; and winds associated with tropical cyclones. The criteria:

Sustained winds	40 miles per hour or greater	last 1 hour or longer
Wind gusts	58 miles per hour or greater	for any duration

Wind Advisory: Issued for the same types of wind events as a High Wind Warning, but at lower speed thresholds. The criteria:

Sustained winds	30 to 39 miles per hour	last one hour or longer
Wind gusts	40 to 57 miles per hour	for any duration

Visibility Hazards: Visibility reduced to a quarter mile or less by fog, blowing dust/sand, and smoke.

Wind Chill: Issued for a wind chill factor of -20 degrees Fahrenheit or colder.

Freezing Rain/Drizzle, or Sleet: widespread, dangerous, and damaging accumulations of ice or sleet.

Frost or Freeze Warning: Issued when temperatures are critical for crops and sensitive plants. Criteria are season dependent, but usually a freeze warning is appropriate when temperatures are expected to fall below freezing for at least two hours.

A new snowy villain we'd never heard of popped up as we completed the first draft of this book in January 2018—a Bomb Cyclone. This is essentially a major cold weather and snow event that acts like a blizzard and hurricane had a baby. A Bomb Cyclone is scientifically known as an explosive cyclogenesis. Some similarities to a hurricane are that this event begins in the ocean, is a low barometric pressure system, and brings high winds to shore. Mix that with bitter record-setting cold, lots of moisture in the form of snow, and you have a recipe for a winter weather disaster.

In the event of any of the above, you can sign up in advance to receive notifications from local emergency services and the National Weather Service, FEMA, the American Red Cross, and other organizations that have free apps which provide up-to-date information about shelters, first aid, and recovery assistance.

Preparation

Warning Fatigue

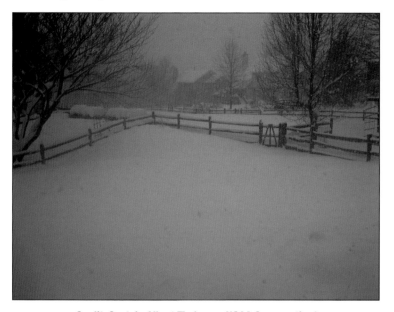

Credit: Captain Albert Theberge, NOAA Corps, retired.

Think of all the warnings you get on a daily or even a weekly basis. Terrorism alerts, security alerts on your computer, fraud alerts for your credit card, smog alerts, and especially, weather alerts for hurricanes, blizzards, high wind, or tornadoes. Because the sheer number of alerts that numb us, the frequency of certain alerts or that we have seen so many "alerts" not come to fruition. We get warning fatigue. This is an age-old problem with weather forecasting. But how do you properly inform the public of the possible dangers without causing this warning fatigue (and subsequent ignoring of the warning)? How long a lead time do you take to begin informing the public of possible weather doom? Meteorologists want the public to take preventative measures, but if they hear and see so many warning alerts and rarely does anything affect them directly, they will more than likely become numb to the warnings.

Blizzards and extreme cold weather events are subject to warning fatigue for sure. The nightly news begins warning a week before icy cold weather is heading your way. That's scary stuff, so you prepare. You anticipate. And nothing much happens. This happens with hurricanes and tornadoes too. Which leads you to say:

"It might affect some but it won't affect me."

"Those guys are hardly ever right."

"We rode out the last one, we can do it again."

Blizzards are the ultimate bad boy storms of cold weather events. If your city or town is in imminent danger of a very heavy snowfall or blizzard, most likely your local weather and news media have let you know in plenty of time. They will be issuing warnings and alerts and, again, these should be taken seriously.

Planning

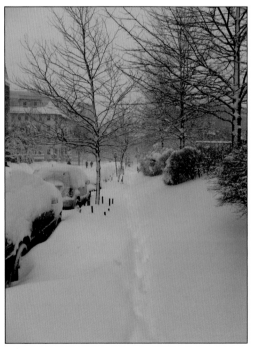

Credit: John Cloud, NOAA Central Library, Washington, DC.

The first step is to create a Family Communications Plan. Two scenarios that can occur: first, your family is together when the blizzard hits whether in the home or on the road; or second, your family is apart. If your family is not together when the blizzard or extreme cold strikes, it is important to know how you will contact one another, how you will all get back together, and what each of you will do in case of an emergency.

Ice storms and blizzards often down power lines and cause havoc to utilities, traffic, and civil services. Prepare for power outages and blocked roads. Shelter, warmth, food, water, and overall safety are your biggest concerns during these cold weather events. Create a supply list of things you will need. Do you know how you will maintain heat if the power goes out? You'd be surprised by how many folks don't realize that their heating system depends on a boiler that is powered by electricity.

So if the power goes out, that means that gas and electric stoves, microwaves, and central heat will not work. You will need to be prepared with alternative heat sources and plenty of blankets. You may have to use candles but you will have to reduce risk of fire, so whenever possible, use battery-powered emergency lights. If your water supply depends on an electric pump, have plenty of bottled water stored somewhere as well.

You might get snowed in, so stock up on snow shovels and snow-removal equipment before any severe snowstorm. Cover the spaces around the doors with weather stripping and cover your windows with stripping as well to keep drafts out, especially if you lose heat. If you get frequent snow events each winter, purchase an appropriate emergency generator, which as an alternate source of power can be a lifesaver. In snowy climes, you'll probably already have a snowplow or snow blower, so make sure to service it regularly.

You may have to dress in layers to thwart the cold. Think big and airy so each layer will trap warm air in. You'll want a supply of warm clothes for each person in the house. If the lights go out, you'll want to find them quickly and easily so keep these items all together in one spot.

Talk with your family about what to do if a winter storm watch or warning is issued. Young children need to hear about the storms to help quell fears and debunk myths. Keep cars and other vehicles fueled and serviced, with a winter emergency kit in each. Be prepared to evacuate if you lose power or heat and know your routes and destinations. Find a local emergency shelter. Check your emergency supplies and individual kits (for the car) and replenish any items missing or in short supply, especially medications and medical supplies.

Know how the public is warned (siren, radio, TV, or app) and the warning terms for each kind of disaster in your community. A winter storm or blizzard warning is timelier than just a watch. While the classifications for conditions are the same as a winter storm watch, a warning means that these conditions are expected within the next twelve hours or sooner.

When a winter storm warning is issued there is little or no time for preparations and as a result, so safety is harder to ensure. When the below warning terms are issued, follow these instructions:

Winter storm watch: Be alert, a storm is likely. Winter weather conditions are expected to cause significant inconveniences and may be hazardous. When caution is used, these situations should not be life threatening. The NWS issues a winter weather advisory when conditions are expected to cause significant inconveniences that may be hazardous. If caution is used, these situations should not be life-threatening.

A winter storm is possible in your area. Tune in to NOAA Weather Radio, commercial radio, or television for more information. The NWS issues a winter storm watch when severe winter conditions, such as heavy snow and/or ice, may affect your area but the location and timing are still uncertain. A winter storm watch is issued twelve to thirty hours in advance of a potential severe storm. Tune in to NOAA Weather Radio, local radio, TV, or other news sources for more information. Monitor alerts, check your emergency supplies, and gather any items you may need if you lose power.

Winter storm warning: Take action as the storm is in or entering the area.

Blizzard warning: Snow and strong winds combined will produce blinding snow, near zero visibility, deep drifts, and life-threatening conditions. Sustained winds or frequent gusts to 35 miles per hour or greater and considerable amounts of falling or blowing snow (reducing visibility to less than a quarter mile) are expected to prevail for a period of three hours or longer.

Wind chill: Seek refuge immediately.

Winter weather advisory: Winter weather conditions are expected to cause significant inconveniences and may be hazardous, especially to motorists.

Frost/freeze warning: Below freezing temperatures are expected and may cause damage to plants, crops, or fruit trees.

Winter Storm Watch: Issued when wintry weather conditions are expected in the next twelve to forty-eight hours. This watch can be upgraded to a blizzard watch when snow and wind gusts of at least 35 miles per hour will drop visibility to less than a quarter mile for three hours or longer.

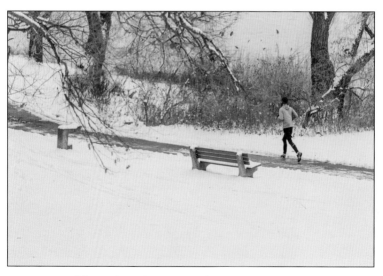

A jogger in a winter storm. *Credit: Matthew Henry.*

Freezing Rain: Rain that freezes when it hits the ground, creating a coating of ice on roads, walkways, trees, and power lines. Take extreme caution when outside.

Sleet: Rain that turns to ice pellets before reaching the ground. Sleet also causes moisture on roads to freeze and become slippery. Take caution when outside.

Each person in your family should know several safe routes from home, work, and school to high ground. Each should know how to contact other household members through a common out-of-state contact in the event you are separated or must evacuate. Know ahead of time what you should do to help elderly or disabled friends, neighbors or employees. If you want to volunteer to help in a disaster, now is the time to sign up with voluntary organizations or the emergency services offices. We advise you do the following:

- Winterize your house, barn, shed, or any other structure that may provide shelter for your family, neighbors, livestock, or equipment.

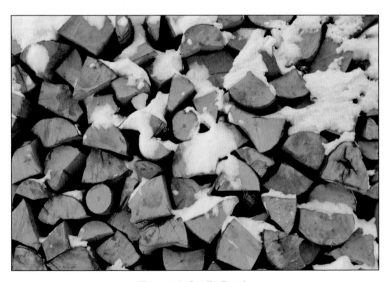

Firewood. *Credit: Pexels.*

- Install storm shutters, doors, and windows.
- Clear rain gutters; repair roof leaks.
- Check the structural ability of the roof to sustain unusually heavy weight from the accumulation of snow—or water (as the snow melts).
- Know how to turn off gas, electric power, and water before evacuating.
- Insulate pipes, valves, and lines.
- Keep plywood, plastic sheeting, lumber, sandbags, and hand tools on hand and accessible.
- Be sure you have ample heating fuel. If you have alternative heating sources, such as fireplaces, wood- or coal-burning stoves, consider buying emergency heating equipment, such as a wood- or coal-burning stove or kerosene heater. Remember to keep all heat sources at least three feet away from furniture and drapes.
- Check that your fire extinguisher(s) is in good working order, and replace it if necessary.
- Bring your companion animals inside and ensure that your horses and livestock have blankets if appropriate and unimpeded access to shelter, food, and non-frozen water.
- Learn how to protect your pipes from freezing.
- Electric space heaters, either portable or fixed. Plug a heater directly into the wall socket rather than using an extension cord and unplug it when it is not in use. Use electric space heaters with automatic shut-off switches and non-glowing elements. If these are relics you got from your grandparents, they aren't probably up to code, and probably aren't safe.
- Consider storing sufficient heating fuel. Regular fuel sources may be cut off. Be cautious of fire hazards when storing any type of fuel.
- If you have a fireplace, consider keeping a supply of firewood or coal. Be sure the fireplace is properly vented and in good working order and that you dispose of ashes safely.

- Make sure you have a working carbon monoxide detector.
- Keep fire extinguishers on hand, and make sure everyone in your house knows how to use them. House fires pose an additional risk, as more people turn to alternate heating sources without taking the necessary safety precautions.

Branches weighed down by heavy, wet snow can become fallen limbs or even downed trees. Saw them into manageable pieces for safe and easy removal—and in some instances, firewood use.

If you have cell phones, make sure each is charged and easy to find. Now is the time to add emergency numbers and apps for easy access when you need them.

Be aware of the potential for flooding when snow and ice melt and be sure that your animals have access to high ground.

Snow may be pretty, but it's still just frozen water. If the temps warm up and that snow starts melting, you could end up with a flooded basement. Meanwhile, you could lose power and your sump pump with it. A battery backup sump pump is your basement's best friend because it's there all the time, especially when you lose power and need it the most.

Traveling in a blizzard is just not a good idea. If you are on the road during a blizzard, look for a hotel or motel nearby and stay off the road until driving conditions are safe again.

However tempting it may be for kids to go out and make snow angels or play in the falling snow, use caution. Those blowing winds—both before and after a blizzard—are cold enough to cause frostbite, and snow drifts may hide dangers children might otherwise not see. Stay indoors where it's safe, and warm.

In many locales, when the weatherperson mentions the possibility of snowfall, grocery stores are swamped. You can't always have perishables like milk, eggs, and bread in your house, so you'll have to slug it out in the grocery store for Grade A eggs with all the other blizzard-worriers, but you can keep many any nonperishables in your house.

Supplies:

Stock your blizzard survival kit with the following:

Water: Power outages will disrupt your water supply if pumps won't operate. Any flooding can contaminate your water supply. So you should have plenty of clean drinking water on hand at all times. It's a good idea to have extra water on hand for washing and food preparation. And throw in a gallon container of water to flush your toilet if the water is off.

Food. For each person, you need to store at least three days' worth of non-perishable food. It won't do you any good if it has to be refrigerated and the power goes out for a week, so make sure to have crackers, cereal, cans of food, peanut butter, dry and canned soup, and the like on hand. Don't forget to include a non-electric can opener in a drawer. Remember to store basic needs for pets and small children.

Flashlights. Have numerous flashlights and battery-powered lanterns. Head lamps are perfect if the lights go out. Have on hand plenty of batteries of all sizes too and make sure they are fresh. A hand-cranked flashlight works when none of the others work.

Power. Do you have a generator? Be prepared to go without electricity for several days, at least. A gas-powered generator selected to meet your needs might keep you warm during the bitter cold. If you have electric-only heat, how will you keep your home warm? Many gas-heated homes need electricity, too. And using a grill or gas stove for heat can prove deadly since both create carbon monoxide fumes.

Medical. Anyone in your family who has need of prescription medicine should stock up before they run out. Always have enough on hand to cover for extended power outages because drugstores and pharmacies may be closed. Have a medical kit in the house that you have supplemented with bandages, antibiotic ointment, aspirin, ibuprofen or other analgesics, antihistamines in case of an allergy attack or an insect bite, and a bottle of alcohol to clean wounds.

Wood. If all else fails, a wood fire will provide warmth. If you have a fireplace, make sure the chimney is in shape, inspected, and ready to go. Have plenty of dry wood on hand, because you'll likely be burning more than you anticipate.

List

- Candles, matches, and lighters.
- Canned foods, non-perishable.
- Freeze-dried non-perishable foods. Other non-perishables (peanut butter, saltines, breakfast bars).
- Non-electric can opener.
- Backup phone chargers.
- Emergency heat sources (fireplaces or wood- or coal-burning stoves) and firewood (if you have a fireplace).
- Rock salt and salt-spreader for driveway and outside walkways (some use sand or non-clumping kitty litter on sidewalks).
- Snow shovel (two if you have other hands on deck).
- Fire extinguisher.
- Flashlights and extra batteries (headlamps come in handy)
- Fuel-powered lanterns or an LED lantern.
- Battery-powered NOAA Weather Radio and portable radio (and preferably a hand-cranked radio, too).
- First aid supplies, medicine and baby items (include aspirin, antacids, band aids, first-aid cream, compress, cold medicines, moleskin).
- Heating fuel (stored smartly).
- Personal medications and items (extra pair of old glasses, prescriptions, hearing aids with extra batteries, glasses, contact lenses, syringes, etc.).
- Multi-purpose tool, other tools you might need.
- Sanitation and personal hygiene items.

- Copies of personal documents (medication list and pertinent medical information, proof of address, deed/lease to home, passports, birth certificates, insurance policies).
- Family and emergency contact information.
- Extra cash (the ATMs may not be working if the power is off).
- Baby supplies (bottles, formula, baby food, diapers).
- Pet supplies (collar, leash, ID, food, carrier, bowl).
- Warm coats, gloves or mittens, hats, boots, and extra blankets and warm clothing for all household members.
- Chainsaw for cutting fallen or hanging limbs (but only if you know what you're doing).

Count on the power being out for at least a day or two and have some board games and a deck of cards on hand. Arts and crafts are always fun for the kids.

If possible, bring your pets inside during cold winter weather. If the animals are outside, make sure their shelters have heat, and their access to food and water is not blocked by snow drifts, ice, or other obstacles. But you really should figure out a way for them to come inside, even if it's in a laundry room or garage. Outside in a blizzard or snowstorm is no place for a pet.

Before the arrival of the snowstorm, protect your pipes from freezing by draining water from swimming pool and water sprinkler supply lines, and water hoses. Add insulation to attics, basements, and crawl spaces. Check around your house for other water supply lines in unheated areas. Insulate water pipes with a pipe sleeve or heat tape or cable. When the weather gets very cold outside, let the cold water drip from the faucet served by exposed pipes. Running water through the pipe, even a trickle, helps prevent pipes from freezing. If you will be going away during cold weather, leave the heat on in your home, set to a temperature no lower than 55° F.

Driving in Snowstorm Conditions

Winter weather, surprisingly, catches communities unprepared. Researchers say that 70 percent of the fatalities related to ice and snow

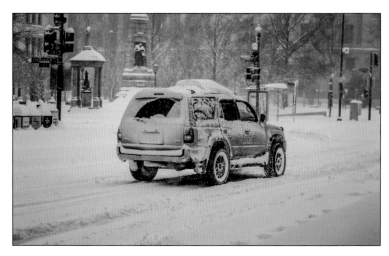

Driving in snowstorms is dangerous. Take extreme caution. *Credit: Pixabay.*

occur in automobiles, and about 25 percent of all winter-related fatalities are people caught off guard, out in the storm.

Have your vehicle winterized before the winter storm season to decrease your chance of being stranded in cold weather. Have a mechanic check your battery, antifreeze, wipers and windshield washer fluid, ignition system, thermostat, lights, flashing hazard lights, exhaust system, heater, brakes, defroster, and oil. Install good winter tires with adequate tread. All-weather radials are usually adequate but some jurisdictions require vehicles to be equipped with chains or snow tires with studs.

Before you go out, you need to have a good reason. If there are blizzard conditions, you simply can't go out. Stay in and be safe. But if the storm hasn't fully hit, if you are traveling out of harm's way, if you have to run up to the store, or pick up a friend for safety's sake, whatever your good reason may be, choose to depart during daylight. If possible, take at least one other person with you. Let someone know your destination, your route, and when you expect to arrive. If your vehicle gets stuck along the way, help can be sent along your predetermined route. Before leaving, listen to weather reports for your area and the areas you will be passing through, or call the state highway patrol for the latest road conditions.

Dress warmly. We've all known someone who wears pajama bottoms and slippers to drive to the store or through a drive-through fast food joint. But what if the car slid off the road? What if they got in a fender bender? Got stuck in the snow?

Be on the lookout for sleet, freezing rain, freezing drizzle, and dense fog, which can make driving very hazardous. Use major streets or highways for travel whenever possible as these roadways will be cleared first.

Drive slowly. Posted speed limits are for ideal weather conditions. Vehicles, including those with four-wheel drive, take longer to stop on snow and ice than on dry pavement. If you skid, steer in the direction you want the car to go and straighten the wheel when the car moves in the desired direction. Try to keep your vehicle's gas tank as full as possible. If you get stuck on the road, stay with your car and contact a towing company.

A majority of ice and snow deaths happen inside of automobiles. When stuck in a vehicle during a blizzard, people should roll the window down a little to allow fresh air inside. This reduces the risk of being poisoned by deadly carbon monoxide gas. Before running the engine, experts recommend checking to make sure the exhaust pipe is not blocked.

If you get stuck and need warmth, the engine can be kept running at ten-minute intervals for warmth. A better idea is to run the engine in short bursts. Turn the engine on long to keep the car warm and then turn it off. Keep this routine up until the conditions are stable enough for you to get back on the road.

Keep these things in your vehicle:

- A windshield scraper, small broom, de-icing spray.
- A small bag of sand for generating traction under the tires.
- A set of tire chains or traction mats.
- Matches in a waterproof container, a couple of lighters.
- A brightly colored (preferably red) cloth to tie to the antenna.
- An emergency supply kit, including warm clothing.
- Keep your vehicle's gas tank full so you can leave right away in an emergency and to keep the fuel line from freezing.

That's hard to do of course, but make it a policy to keep your fuel at half-full during winter.

- Keep a supply of kitty litter to make walkways and steps less slippery.
- Make sure you have a cell phone with an emergency charging option (car, solar, hand crank, etc.) in case your car gets stuck or loses power.
- Blanket or two.
- Flashlights with extra batteries.
- Small supply of non-perishable food.
- Shovel.
- Tool kit.
- Jumper cables.
- Road maps (cell service may not work).
- Flares.

Survival

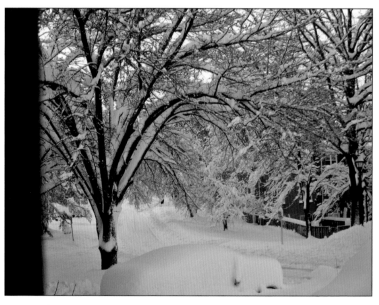

Snowmageddon in Gaithersburg, Maryland, February 6, 2010.
Credit: Kevin Shaw, NOAA, NOS, OCS.

You've had plenty of warning about the impending storm. Do you stay or do you go? If you have time to drive, as long as it's with good visibility, away from the storm not into it, and with a destination where you can stay a good while if the storm shuts down your community, then perhaps you should leave. But let's assume you end up staying in your house, which is the only way to ensure survival. Avoid the blizzard by staying in and remaining warm.

Stay inside. Keep the heat set in the mid-sixties during the day and cooler even at night to conserve fuel. Shut off unneeded rooms to save heat. Cover the windows at night. Eat and drink to prevent dehydration. Wear layers of loose-fitting, lightweight, and warm clothing around the house. Do not drive until it's safe to do so.

If the power goes out, do not heat your home with stoves or charcoal grills. These heaters release carbon monoxide, and it can poison you without you even knowing because it's a colorless and odorless gas. Monitor your NOAA Weather Radio and keep a local radio and/or TV station on for information and emergency instructions. Have your emergency survival kit ready to go if told to evacuate. Know where the manual release lever of your electric garage door opener is located and how to operate it in case you lose power.

Keep food as safe as possible. Keep the refrigerator and freezer doors closed and don't open them unless you're getting food out and do it quickly. First, eat the perishable food from the refrigerator. An unopened refrigerator will keep foods cold for about four hours. After that's gone, use the food from the freezer. A full freezer will keep its temperature for about forty-eight hours, but only if the door remains closed. Eat your non-perishable foods and staples after using food from the refrigerator and freezer.

If it looks like the power outage will continue for more than a day, prepare a cooler with ice for your freezer items. Keep food in a dry, cool spot and keep it covered at all times. Turn off and unplug all unnecessary electrical equipment, including sensitive electronics. Turn off or disconnect any appliances (stoves, equipment, or electronics) you were using when the power went out. When power comes back on, you want to avoid surges or spikes since they can damage equipment. Leave a light on so you'll know when the power comes back on.

Before you go outside, dress in layers. The outer layer of your clothes should be waterproof and wind-stopping. Your jacket should have a hood or you should have a head covering (hat, beanie, ear muffs, etc.) Wear mittens or gloves. Wear waterproof, insulated shoes or boots.

If a fallen wire has fallen over a car, don't approach the car to make a rescue attempt. Remain a safe distance away and try to keep the occupant of the vehicle calm. If possible, let emergency personnel handle the situation.

If you must travel during a storm, do so during the day and inform someone of your itinerary, route, and expected arrival time. Stay alert and look out for other cars and rescue teams. If you must go out during a winter storm, use public transportation if possible. About 70 percent of winter deaths related to ice and snow occur in automobiles.

If a Blizzard Traps You in Your Car:

Don't keep driving. Pull off the road, turn on your hazard lights, and hang a distress flag from the radio antenna or window. If the snow piles up around your vehicle, you'll want something above the car alerting rescuers. Remain in your vehicle. Rescuers will look there first. You don't want a drift of snow to block your exhaust. Hopefully, you've prepared for any snowstorm by including a blizzard emergency kit in your car.

A blizzard not only means that you can't see but other cars can't see you until it ends. You can't keep the car running or you'll run out of fuel and freeze. Conserve gas but run the engine and heater about ten minutes each hour to keep warm. Make sure to roll down window ever so slightly to prevent carbon monoxide poisoning. Exercise to maintain body heat but don't overexert. Huddle with other passengers and use your coat for a blanket. In extreme cold, use road maps, seat covers, floor mats, newspapers, or extra clothing to provide additional insulation and warmth.

Do light exercises to keep up circulation. Clap your hands and move your arms and legs occasionally. Don't stay in one position for too long. If more than one person is in the vehicle, take turns sleeping so one can monitor conditions and turn the car on periodically. If not, you could both freeze to death.

Watch for signs of frostbite and hypothermia. Severe cold can cause numbness, making you unaware of possible danger. Avoid overexertion. Cold weather puts an added strain on the heart. Pushing a vehicle, for instance, can bring on a heart attack or make other medical conditions worse.

Don't get out of your car unless you need to use the bathroom and don't set out on foot unless you see a building close by where you know you can take shelter. Once the blizzard is over, you may need to leave the car and proceed on foot. Follow the road if at all possible. If you need to walk across open country, use distant points as landmarks to help maintain your sense of direction.

If Caught Outside During a Blizzard:

You need to get out of the shearing bitter cold winds immediately. Find a dry shelter immediately. Cover all exposed body parts. The blizzard will likely be disorienting so look for landmarks that will lead you to a safehouse or a warm building. Look for a mailbox, a driveway, a parking lot, any kind of physical clue to get to a building.

If you are not in a city or town, but out on a country road or on a long part of a highway and your car is out of gas or is immobilized and won't start, you won't easily find refuge. Now is the time to use your survival skills.

Can you find anything with which to prepare a lean-to, a wind break, or to build a snow-cave for protection against the wind? Any way to build a fire for heat and attention purposes? Is there a stand of trees or thick bushes you can use for protection? If you can, use it.

Frostbite and Hypothermia

Frostbite

Frostbite is a serious condition where parts of your body actually freeze due to not properly being protected in frigid temperatures. Your

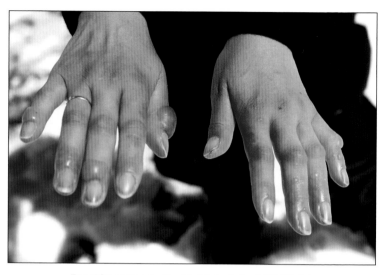

Frostbite on hands. *Credit: Winky Oxford, UK (Flickr),*
creativecommons.org licenses by 2.0.

extremities are at the greatest risk since they are further away from your warmer core. Frostnip, the first stage of frostbite, is when your unprotected skin gets red and sore. Take this signal as a serious warning to bundle up, get inside, and to ward off progression to more serious stages. Frostbite can happen in minutes so there isn't much time to play around with warning signs. Once frostbite begins it's tough to realize how serious the damage is due to lack of feeling, so noticing the color of your skin is telling as to how deep and damaging the frostbite has progressed. When the skin darkens to blue and black, this is the most advanced stage and damage has likely gone all the way to the bone.

First signs include:

- Pins and needles feeling in the skin.
- Skin turns a pale color.

Later signs:
- Skin hardens and takes on a shiny or waxy appearance.
- Blisters form as skin thaws.

More advanced signs:
- Skin turns a dark blue or black color.
- Skin feels cold to touch and is hard.

Seek medical attention quickly if you or anyone you know is experiencing frostbite, especially at the late and advanced stages. If that's not an option right away, then get to a warm place immediately and do not rub the affected skin. Also, soak affected areas in warm, not hot, water or place a warm washcloth over the frostbitten area. As skin thaws you'll feel prickly, stinging feeling coming back to your skin. Keep area covered with a loose, dry dressings and place gauze between toes to keep them separated. Use caution so you don't break any blisters that may have formed.

Frostbite is a bad deal, so do what you can to avoid it:

- Take frequent breaks from the cold.
- Cover your extremities, ears included, with a good hat, gloves, and socks that wick away moisture.
- Wear loose, layered clothing with a first layer of moisture wicking material.
- Dry off if your clothing becomes wet from sweat or snow as wet clothing makes the likelihood of frostbite higher.

Hypothermia

Hypothermia develops when a person's core body temperature falls below 95 degrees Fahrenheit and severe hypothermia develops at a body temperature of 82 degrees Fahrenheit or lower. Hypothermia is usually caused from extended exposure to cold temperatures and that risk increases during the cold, winter months. When exposed to cold temperatures, our bodies lose heat at a faster rate than it can be produced, so staying out for too long in cold temps uses up our body's storehouse of warmth. This lowering of body temperature is a serious condition, so take steps to avoid it, and know how to recognize when it sets in. Note that body temperatures may vary from person to person so stay tuned to all of the signs of hypothermia.

Signs to be aware of:

- Shivering, which helps the body produce heat with muscle activity.
- Weakness, including slow breathing, slow speech, low pulse, drowsiness, and loss of coordination.
- Confusion or apathy.
- Glassy stare.
- Infants may exhibit low energy with cold, bright red skin.
- Most serious cases result in unconsciousness.

If you or someone you know is experiencing signs of hypothermia, seek medical attention and call 911, especially if extreme hypothermia has set in, including when body temperature falls below 95 degrees. In the meantime, get to a warmer location and monitor breathing and circulation. Get into dry, warm clothes and begin warming up slowly with blankets and possibly heating pads or electric blankets applied to core body areas. Keep from warming the body too quickly; warm the core (midsection) first. Try drinking warm liquids, but not alcohol or caffeine.

If the affected person is unconscious, again, call for medical help right away. If there is no pulse or sign of breathing, immediately begin CPR (make sure there is no pulse before starting CPR; this may take a bit to know since the heart rate is likely slow). Once CPR is the course of action, keep it up until medical help arrives or breathing or a pulse has been restored. Remember that confusion can set in, making the affected person's ability to make good decisions for their safety difficult.

Hypothermia is a scary situation, so take precautions to avoid it.

- Make note of the temperature, including wind chill, and don't stay in the cold too long; if necessary, take breaks inside.
- Dress accordingly by covering exposed skin and dressing in loose, warm layers with water wicking layers closest to the skin.
- Stay hydrated with warm fluids, excluding alcohol and caffeine, and eat high-fat carbs.

- Stay moving to keep your core warm.
- Take extra precautions with infants, children, elderly, and with those who have conditions that increase hypothermia risk (diabetes, thyroid conditions, or use of drugs or alcohol).

If you experience any signs, get inside and get warm.

Carbon Monoxide Caution: Each year, more than four hundred Americans die from unintentional carbon monoxide poisoning, and there are more than twenty thousand visits to the emergency room with more than four thousand hospitalizations. Carbon monoxide-related deaths are highest during colder months, likely due to increased use of gas-powered furnaces and alternative heating, cooking, and power sources used inappropriately indoors during power outages.

- Never use a generator, grill, camp stove, or other gasoline, propane, natural gas, or charcoal-burning devices inside a home, garage, basement, or any partially enclosed area. Locate the unit away from doors, windows and vents that could allow carbon monoxide to come indoors. Keep these devices at least twenty feet from doors, windows, and vents.
- The primary hazards to avoid when using alternate sources for electricity, heating, or cooking are carbon monoxide poisoning, electric shock, and fire.
- Install carbon monoxide alarms in central locations on every level of your home and outside sleeping areas to provide early warning of accumulating carbon monoxide.
- If the carbon monoxide alarm sounds, move quickly to a fresh air location outdoors or by an open window or door.
- Call for help from the fresh air location and remain there until emergency personnel arrive to assist you.

Aftermath

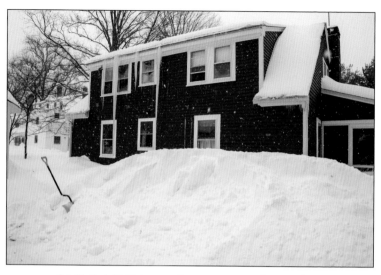

Credit: Dwight Sipler, creativecommons.org.licenses.b.2.0.

Just because the blizzard or big snow event has passed doesn't mean you are out of the woods yet. You may have lost power to your house and be without adequate heat. The streets may be impassable with drifts or heavy snow or ice. Your car may be buried under snow. Power lines may be downed and causing dangers on the roads or yards. The temperatures may still be cold enough to cause frostbite or hypothermia. The sidewalks and driveway may be icy and slick so that even walking to your car is dangerous.

If your home loses power or heat for more than a few hours or if you do not have adequate supplies to stay warm in your house overnight, it might be time to consider going to a designated public shelter. Text **SHELTER** + your **ZIP code** to **43362** (4FEMA) to find the nearest shelter in your area (e.g., SHELTER20472).

If you find yourself in a shelter, it's going to be odd sleeping in an open space with so many other people of differing nighttime habits. Bring ear plugs for starters. Bring any personal items that you need (toiletries, medicines) but only bring what you need for a night or two.

Dress warmly so that if you have only a blanket, you're still warm. If you bring a phone and charger, and you should, don't leave it charging without you being able to see it. Better safe than sorry. Eat to maintain calories and warmth and stay indoors as much as possible.

If you are able to stay in your home, take inventory of damage in and around your house. Report downed power lines and broken gas lines immediately. Is there damage to your roof? Your water pipes? If you have a chimney, check it to be sure it has no structural damage. And if you light a fire, be sure the smoke does not back up into your home.

Repair broken windows by covering them with plywood or taping blankets or tarps over them to offer some insulation until a repair person can provide proper repair. If the house sustained structural damage, stay with a neighbor if you can.

Don't let children or pets run around outside without knowing if there are downed lines. Check for any leaks in your ceiling as they could mean roof damage. Check for broken tree limbs. Limbs could fall damage your yard, auto, home, or worse, even cause potential injury to someone underneath.

If there are no other problems, wait for streets and roads to be opened before you attempt to drive anywhere.

Check on neighbors, especially any who might need help.

You may be tempted to shovel your walks and driveway. Beware of overexertion and exhaustion. Because you could hurt your back, overexert yourself, and have a heart attack, why not use a snow blower instead? If you don't have one, perhaps a kindly neighbor will clear your paths or perhaps it's time to pay a small amount to a local service to do it.

But you are stubborn and you want to shovel snow yourself. Hopefully, you bought an ergonomic shovel with a curved or adjustable handle. Don't go out in the cold with cold muscles. Warm up and stretch your muscles especially your lower back and hamstrings. Don't lift the snow if you can help it but push it to the side. Stay square, bend at the hips, keep loads light, avoid twisting, and grip one hand near the load. Most importantly, pace yourself, don't overexert. Keep good footing so you don't slip and fall. Take a break every few minutes. Don't start sweating underneath your layers of clothes.

The streets may be tall with snowdrifts. Sidewalks may be slick with ice. Your car may be buried. Side streets won't be frequently traveled and will be treacherous, so stay on main thoroughfares. Keep listening to a local station on battery-powered radio or television or to NOAA Weather Radio for updated emergency information. You may be in for more snow so stay informed.

Eat regularly. Food provides your body with energy to produce its own heat. Replenish your body with fluids to prevent dehydration. Avoid caffeine and alcohol since caffeine, a stimulant, accelerates the symptoms of hypothermia. Alcohol is a depressant and hurries the effects of cold on the body. Both caffeine and alcohol can cause dehydration. Throw out unsafe food. Throw away any food that has been exposed to temperatures above freezing for two hours or more or if it has an unusual odor, color, or texture. When in doubt, throw it out.

Conserve fuel. Winter storms can place great demand on electric, gas, and other fuel distribution systems. Keep your thermostats lowered to 65 degrees Fahrenheit during the day and 55 degrees Fahrenheit at night. Close off rooms you are not using. Cover the cracks under the doors.

If you turn on a faucet and only a trickle comes out, you probably have a frozen pipe. These typically occur against exterior walls or entry points for the water service. Keep the faucet open. Apply heat to the section of pipe using a hair dryer, a heating pad, even a space heater but don't use a blowtorch, kerosene or propane heater, charcoal stove, or other open flame device.

As you treat the frozen pipe and the frozen area begins to melt, water should flow through the frozen area. Water running through the pipe will help melt ice in the pipe. If you are unable to locate the frozen area, if the frozen area is not accessible, or if you cannot thaw the pipe, call a licensed plumber. You don't want broken pipes and resultant flooding.

CHAPTER SEVEN

LANDSLIDES AND MUDSLIDES

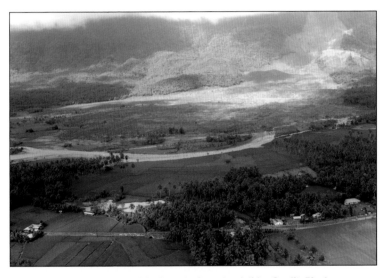

Aerial view of the Philippines during a landslide. *Credit: Pixabay.*

Landslides don't seem like they would occur often enough that you should even worry about preparation or survival. On average, between twenty-five and fifty people are reported killed by landslides in America, although the real numbers exceed that amount because many landslide and debris flow deaths are attributed to the catalyst such as earthquakes.

While the California landslides make the most headlines, landslides occur in almost every state and can cause significant damage. The states considered most vulnerable are Washington, Oregon, California, Alaska, and Hawaii. The term landslide describes downhill earth movements that can move slowly and cause damage gradually, or move rapidly, destroying property and taking lives suddenly and unexpectedly.

A landslide is a large mass of earth and rocks that suddenly slides down the side of a hill, slope, or mountain. You'll also hear landslides referred to as debris flows, mudslides, mudflows, or debris avalanches. Landslides are dangerous because they happen in a flash, move at extremely high speeds, and they are able to travel long distances.

Landslides occur from human, structural, or geological forces but most landslides are caused by natural events, such as heavy rain, snowmelt, earthquakes, volcanic eruptions, erosion, change in ground water, and gravity. If the force down-slope exceeds the strength of the earth materials below, you get a landslide.

Human influences that cause landslides include mining, logging, irrigation, and excavation. Landslides are typically associated with periods of heavy rainfall or rapid snowmelt and tend to worsen the effects of flooding by adding debris. Areas of land that are degraded by fire are vulnerable to landslides. One important thing to know: Landslides typically happen in areas where they have happened before. So that means you need to learn about your area's landslide risk.

Landslide problems can be caused by land mismanagement, particularly in mountain, canyon, and coastal regions. In areas burned by forest and brush fires, a lower threshold of precipitation may initiate landslides.

Impending landslide warning signs:

- Springs, seeps, or saturated ground in areas that have not typically been wet before.

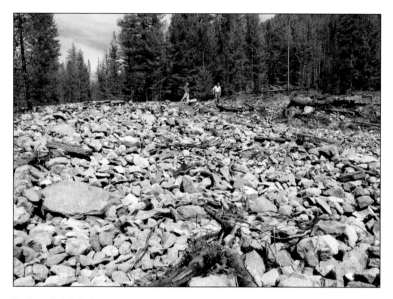

Badger Gulch in Beavercreek, Idaho after wildfire and heavy rainfall. *Credit: US Geological Survey, creativecommons.org licenses by 2.0, Wikimedia Commons.*

- New cracks or unusual bulges in the ground, street pavements, or sidewalks.
- Soil moving away from foundations.
- Ancillary structures such as decks and patios tilting and/or moving relative to the main house.
- Tilting or cracking of concrete floors and foundations.
- Broken water lines and other underground utilities.
- Leaning telephone poles, trees, retaining walls, or fences.
- Offset fence lines.
- Sunken or down-dropped road beds.
- Rapid increase in creek water levels, possibly accompanied by increased turbidity (soil content).
- Sudden decrease in creek water levels though rain is still falling or just recently stopped.
- Sticking doors and windows, and visible open spaces indicating jambs and frames out of plumb.
- A faint rumbling sound that increases in volume is noticeable as the landslide nears.

- Unusual sounds, such as trees cracking or boulders knocking together, might indicate moving debris.

Preparation

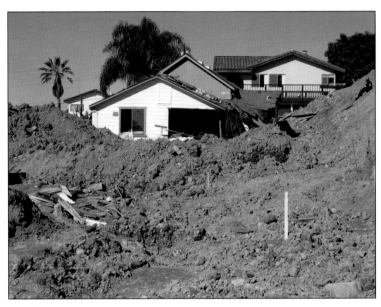

California homes after a damaging landslide.
Credit: John Shea, FEMA Photo Library.

So what can you do to protect yourself and your property from a landslide?

If you haven't built your home yet, research before you build your house. Has this area experienced landslides or debris flows in the past? Are there water drainage patterns where runoff converges and causes channels, natural indicators of landslides? Do you see erosion valleys? If you want to build near steep slopes or close to a mountain's edge, your builder should do a ground assessment and provide necessary information about possible landslides.

If you have a house in place, assess your property's landslide risk. There are various ways to do this—get in touch with local officials, local universities (geology), state geological surveys, natural resource departments and get a ground assessment of your property. Ask for information on landslides in your area, request specific information on areas vulnerable to landslides, and get a professional referral for a detailed site analysis of your property, and what you can do to correct the situation if possible.

Minimize home hazards:

- Plant ground cover on slopes.
- Build retaining walls.
- Build deflection walls in mudflow areas so the debris flow goes around your house (but don't force it to a neighbor's lawn or you're responsible).
- Use flexible pipe fittings since they are more resistant to breakage so you avoid gas or water leaks.
- Bring in a professional to consult on preventative action.

Watch for clues: Are you on or near a steep slope? Close to the edge of a mountain? In a natural erosion zone? Do you see any patterns after rain

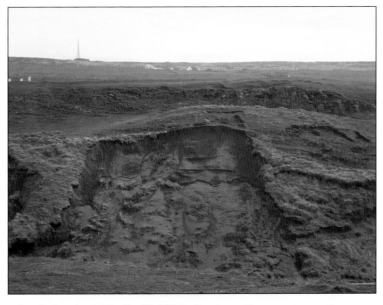

Small slope landslide. *Credit: Eddylandzaat, creativecommons.org licenses by-sa 3.0 nl deed.en, Wikimedia Commons.*

where runoff water converges and forms heavy channels? Do you see any new changes in your landscape that are probably the result of drainage? Any land movement or small slides? Leaning trees? Are there new cracks that have appeared in the ground, your driveway, side of your foundation? Is your fence leaning more after rains? Have debris flows occurred in your area before? All of these could indicate that you are in danger of a possible landslide occurrence on your property.

No single indicator should alert you that landslides are possible or imminent but there are a collection of signs to watch for: Look for warping in your home or movement in the area near your home. Take

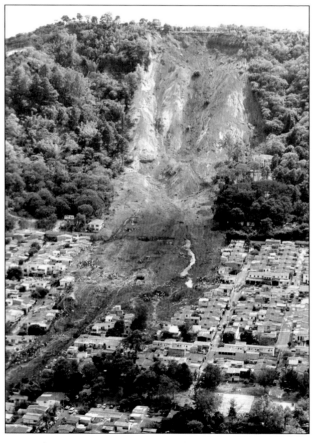

A devastating landslide in El Salvador. *Credit: USGS.*

note if your deck, patio, or concrete floors are tilting, pulling away from the building, or cracking. If your doors and windows are sticking, that might indicate warping. Broken water lines, roadbeds that seem to have sunken overnight, cracks in plaster or brick, outside walls that are pulling away, and widening cracks in pavement should all be causes for concerns. Do you have any underground utility lines that have broken? Any bulging ground that appears at the base of a slope? Any water breaking through the ground surface in new locations? Do you see any fences, retaining walls, utility poles, or trees tilting or moving? If you live where you could experience a landslide, keep eyes wide open and stay safe.

If your area is vulnerable to landslides, talk to an insurance agent to see if your insurance covers landslide-related damage. Although landslide insurance is not usually available, some flood insurance policies cover damage from landslide flows. To begin preparing, you should build an emergency kit and make a family communications plan.

Buy a NOAA Radio and have it handy. The NOAA Weather Radio is an automated twenty-four-hour network of radio stations in the United States that broadcast advertisement-free weather information directly from a nearby National Weather Service office. If your area is receiving heavy rainfall, check the radio or television station for any landslide warnings or alerts. We recommend also downloading at least one emergency app for iPhone or Android since so many are now available for any disaster. There are several disaster alert apps so find the ones that work for you. Most include interactive maps, alerts, information, contacts and more. Facebook has a Safety Check-in feature that alerts all your friends and family who have already heard about the disaster in your area, that you are safe.

Power could be out or phone systems might be down, but you can use various apps that provide free IM and phone calling. You know how quickly apps come and go, how they are improved or even change names, so it doesn't make sense to list them here when by the time the book comes out, the list would have changed.

Your family might be in different places when a landslide hits, so make sure everyone knows how to receive emergency alerts from local officials, by phone, television, radio, text, or phone app. More and more, emergency updates are provided by text.

Learn about local emergency response and evacuation plans. Landslide-prone areas typically have an emergency response team and evacuation plans. You might consider participating in local emergency response groups. Talk to everyone in your household about what to do if a landslide occurs. Create and practice an evacuation plan for your family and your business.

Additionally, assemble and maintain an emergency preparedness kit and create and practice an evacuation plan for your family and your business.

You will want to write down each family member's phone number, email, all their social media names, doctors' names and medical facilities, medicines, allergies, and school or workplace information. Take a photo with your phone just to have a backup. In the event of a landslide, you need to choose a place where the family will reunite. Pick a location in your neighborhood or at your church or a community center. If you worry about the landslide hitting your entire area, choose a meeting place somewhere central in your town. If you have pets, pick a pet-friendly area. Make sure everyone is aware of that location.

Compile contact information, landslide safety protocol, and your emergency meeting places on a single document. This is your emergency plan. Give every family member a copy and make sure they carry it with them at all times.

Your emergency kit

Each person in the house should have their own emergency kit in case you have to quickly evacuate.

- First-aid kit.
- Several-day supply of medicine.
- Flashlight and extra batteries. Hand-crank flashlight too.
- Battery-powered radio, and a hand-crank radio too.
- Three-day water supply (one gallon per person daily).

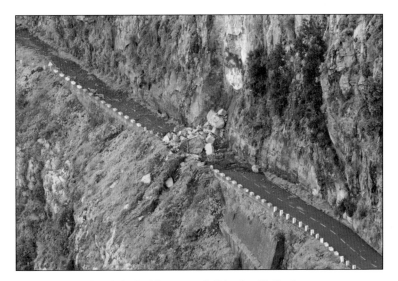

Road blocked from a rockslide. *Credit: Pixabay.*

- Three-day supply of easy-to-store, easy-to-prepare food that stores well such as dried or canned soups, protein bars, canned meat, beef jerky, powdered milk, canned vegetables and fruits, saltines, peanut butter, and hard candy.
- Personal hygiene items,
- Basic tool kit or at least a multi-use tool.
- Contact information of family and emergency departments.
- Ziploc bags for your mobile phones (not a bad idea to have an extra charger).
- Copies of important documents such as birth certificates, passports, insurance policies, proof of address, and the lease or deed to your home.
- Cash and change (ATMs might not be working or have cash left).

If you live in an area known for landslides, your area could be hit by a landslide and even if your house survives, you might be isolated or trapped, so it's a good idea to have an emergency supply kit at your house

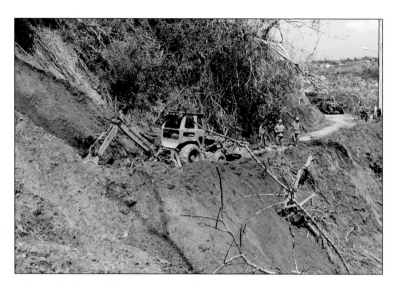

Cleanup in Puerto Rico after a landslide. *Credit: Sgt. Alexis Vélez, Puerto Rico National Guard, Wikimedia Commons.*

with enough food and water to last three days. Landslides can interrupt services such as electricity, gas, water, phones, and sewage so plan accordingly. If your business is located in a landslide-prone area, it makes sense to prepare with the same vigor as you do with your home prep.

Survival

Conditions are prime for a landslide. Now what?

If you suspect imminent landslide danger, you've assessed the situation, and you are fairly sure a landslide is about to happen, contact your local fire, police, or public works department. Local officials are the best persons able to assess potential danger. Talk to your neighbors who might be in danger, too. They may not know of the potential threat and there may be some who need help evacuating. After you've done your due diligence, leave. Evacuate. Your best bet for your safety is to not be in the way of the landslide.

You might be at home, at work, or out of town but if you are in the middle of a severe storm and are in a landslide zone, pay attention. If

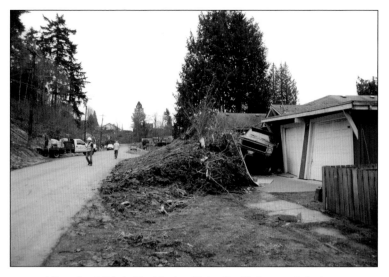

After a landslide in Washington State. *Credit: Savannah Brehmer, FEMA Photograph Library.*

an earthquake just occurred near your area and you are in the path of a possible landslide (streamside, slope, or mountain), pay attention.

It's raining heavily—a real gully washer—and you are concerned about a landslide. What do you do? During a severe storm, stay alert and awake. Many deaths from landslides occur while people are sleeping. Here's your list of things to watch and listen for: turn on the NOAA radio and your local television station; unusual sounds, such as trees cracking or boulders knocking together; a low rumbling sound, which might indicate moving debris; collapsed pavement, new mud, falling rocks; roadside embankments caving in; earthquakes, which can induce or intensify the effects of landslides.

If you are with other people during the night and worrying about a possible landslide, coordinate your efforts and work together to keep each other awake. The alert parties should listen to the local news for updates on evacuation or impending landslide. If the weather is not too severe to travel, then why take the risk? You and your family should evacuate whether or not the emergency management team has ordered it.

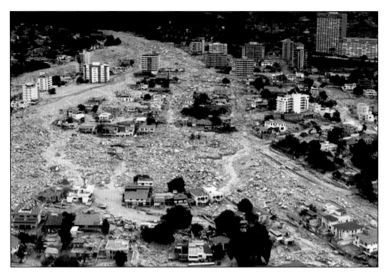

Tragic debris flow after heavy rains and flooding in Vargas, Venezuela.
Credit: John Shea, USGS. FEMA Photo Library.

Steps toward evacuation

- Listen to local and/or NOAA radio or watch local TV for warnings about intense rainfall or for information and instructions from local officials.
- Be aware that a trickle of mud or debris slowly moving or falling may precede a larger landslide.
- If you have a stream nearby, watch for any dramatic change in water level, up or down, clarity turning muddy. The landslide/mud debris could be occurring way upstream and you could see indicators well before it arrives.
- If you've decided it's worth leaving your house, grab your emergency kits, and drive with a watchful eye. Watch for any tall structure that is unusually tilting or falling such as fences, trees or utility poles. As you look around, are there any big bald spots on hills or mountains around you, places where a landslide might have occurred already?

- As you drive, be alert. We've driven on mountain roads that became blocked by a mud/landslide or closed by collapsed pavement right before we got there. Try to avoid low-lying areas or river valleys.
- Bridges could be washed out.
- Do not cross flooding streams. Turn Around, Don't Drown.

The Landslide is Happening

You've seen the landslide and mudslide videos before and know that folks will stand on the side of the flow watching it disbelievingly rush past them. Don't do that. Move to higher ground immediately. Those folks are in danger of that ground being swept up in the forceful erosion of the slide.

Cracking trees and breaking boulders are a sign that a landslide is upon you. Run to high ground immediately.

If you get swept up in a landslide/mudslide, your potential for survival is small, some experts say less than 10 percent. Caught in the slurry of a slide makes swimming next to impossible and the quickness and force of the debris flow can knock you unconscious or injure your body. Your best bet is to either try to climb out, climb on top of something floating or something solid to grab ahold of. But it's a small chance—so don't get caught in a landslide!

Aftermath

The landslide has rushed past you or within a block or two of you. Perhaps you got to high ground but your house is demolished. Or maybe you avoided the catastrophe but are blocked in by debris. You might even be loading up the station wagon to leave the area. What should you do next? Avoid the area where the landslide occurred. Don't be an onlooker unless you are part of a local emergency response team. Landslides may recur in the same location, so avoid this area and seek shelter.

After a landslide has passed, you should remain in a safe place until authorities have announced it is safe to leave. Listen to the radio for

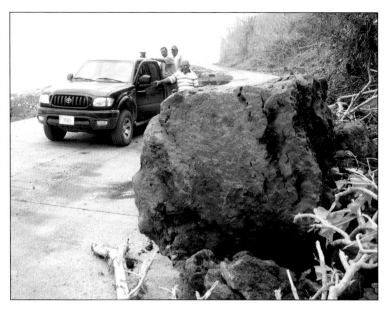

Boulder sits at rest on side of the road after a dangerous slide.
Credit: Barry Markowitz, FEMA Photo Library.

emergency updates. When you decide to go out, stay alert for flooding, debris, and damage to roads, utilities, and power lines.

Avoid river valleys and other low areas. These areas are especially dangerous when landslides are imminent, so stay away.

Go to a public shelter. Your local community should have a designated public shelter. Go to the shelter if your home is unsafe or the authorities have called for an evacuation. To find the shelter closest to you, text SHELTER + your ZIP code to 43362 (4FEMA). For example, if your zip code is 56789, you would text SHELTER 56789.

Help neighbors who need special assistance. Infants, the disabled, and the elderly may experience extra difficulty in emergency situations. If it is safe to do so, help your neighbors with special needs. Remember that neighbors with large families may require additional assistance as well. If you are in a building, examine its foundation, chimney and surrounding land to determine if the structure is stable. If the area appears unsafe, leave immediately.

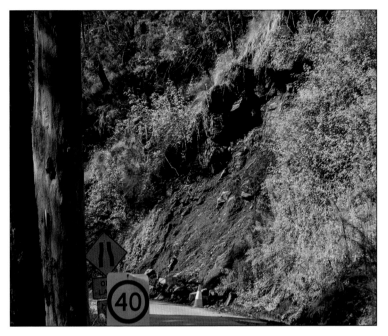

Small landslides occur frequently. *Credit: Pixabay.*

Some additional instructions:

- Stay away from the site. Flooding or additional slides may occur after a landslide or mudflow.
- Listen to the radio or TV for emergency information.
- Report broken utility lines to the appropriate authorities.
- Stay away from the slide area. There may be danger of additional slides.
- Listen to local radio or television stations for the latest emergency information.
- Watch for flooding, which may occur after a landslide or debris flow. Floods sometimes follow landslides and debris flows because they may both be started by the same event.
- Check for injured and trapped persons near the slide, without entering the direct slide area. Direct rescuers to their locations.

- Look for and report broken utility lines and damaged roadways and railways to appropriate authorities. Reporting potential hazards will get the utilities turned off as quickly as possible, preventing further hazard and injury.
- Check the building foundation, chimney, and surrounding land for damage. Damage to foundations, chimneys, or surrounding land may help you assess the safety of the area.
- Replant damaged ground as soon as possible since erosion caused by loss of ground cover can lead to flash flooding and additional landslides in the near future.
- Seek advice from an expert for evaluating landslide hazards and designing corrective techniques to reduce future landslide risk.

CHAPTER EIGHT

FLOODS

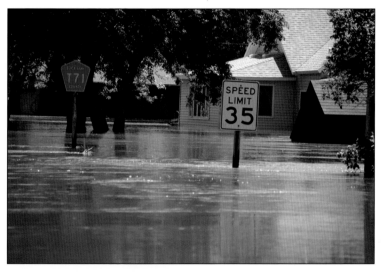

A flooded neighborhood. *Credit: Don Becker, USGS.*

The most common and therefore most dangerous weather disaster event is flooding. Every year, flooding is America's most common natural disaster and destroys communities around the world.

So what is a flood? Flooding may happen with only a few inches of water, or it may rise to rooftop level. There are many possible causes of floods including heavy rain or snowmelt, coastal storms and storm surge, waterway overflow from being blocked with debris or ice, or overflow of levees, dams, or waste water systems. Flooding can occur slowly over many days or happen very quickly with little or no warning. These are called flash floods. One of the most devastating forms of flooding comes from hurricanes hitting land, even as they decay on their inward movement and fill up rivers and lakes. This is because heavy rains are localized and raise river flow in a short amount of time. Flash floods are the result, and unlike many other flood events, these don't provide much warning. In fact, it doesn't take much rain to cause a river to overflow and flood an area. One of the predominant causes of river flash flooding is when a river has blockage (landslide, glacier, dam failure or the like) and the resultant release of built-up water causes catastrophe.

Two key elements that contribute to flooding include rainfall intensity and duration. Intensity is the rate of rainfall and how long it keeps raining. Topography, soil conditions, and ground cover also play important roles in flooding. Don't think that all is bad. Flooding has its good side—natural flooding of river plains and deltas are essential for farming by bringing nutrient-rich soil.

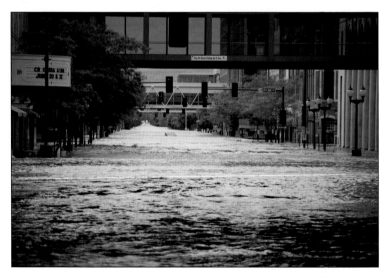

Flooding in Cedar Rapids, Iowa. *Credit: Don Becker, USGS.*

Around the globe, we have built cities along the coast, and three-quarters of the world's megacities lie on the coast. Over 80 percent of our world's population lives within sixty miles of coastal waters and over 50 percent of the world's population lives within closer than half a mile to a freshwater body of water. With most cities and towns located at the coast or next to rivers, flood events can be major natural disasters, causing extensive loss of life and damage to land and property. Flood losses in the United States averaged $2.4 billion per year for the last decade. And over 50 percent of the world's population lives within closer than half a mile to a freshwater body of water. The Yellow River in China has had the four deadliest flood events in world history. Its 1931 floods killed an unbelievable one to four million people. Humankind has always lived close to water and that means existence comes with risks of natural disasters.

Flooding may happen with only a few inches of water, or it may rise to rooftop level. There are many possible causes of floods including heavy rain or snowmelt, coastal storms and storm surge, waterway overflow from being blocked with debris or ice, or overflow of levees, dams, or wastewater systems. Flooding can occur slowly over many days or happen very quickly with little or no warning, called flash floods. One of the most devastating forms of flooding comes from hurricanes hitting land, even as they decay on their inward movement and fill up rivers and lakes.

Urbanization has caused much more flooding today than before. As woodlands and fields are converted to parking lots, roads, and shopping centers, that land can no longer absorb rainfall. That water has to go somewhere and the resultant runoff from urbanization is many times what it would normally be. Your neighborhood or business street is much more likely to become a quick-moving river than ever before.

Floods can damage bridges, roads, and other transportation infrastructure. Infrastructure such as buildings, cars, and houses can be left saturated or completely taken by the waters. Sewage systems and power grids can be destroyed. After floodwaters recede, land can be contaminated with hazardous material, such as building debris, fuel, and untreated sewage. Residents are often left without power or clean drinking water which can lead to outbreaks of diseases.

Most flash flooding is caused by slow-moving thunderstorms, thunderstorms repeatedly moving over the same area, or heavy rains from hurricanes and tropical storms. Floods, on the other hand, can be slow- or fast-rising, but generally develop over a period of hours or days. Flash floods, on the other hand, occur within six hours of a rain event, or after a dam or levee failure, or following a sudden release of water held by an ice or debris jam, and flash floods can catch people unprepared. Because you will not always have a warning that these deadly, sudden floods are coming, plan now to protect your family and property.

Flooding can happen in any US state or territory. It is particularly important to be prepared for flooding if you live in a low-lying area near a body of water, such as near a river, stream, or culvert, along a coast, or downstream from a dam or levee. Flooding can occur during every season, but some areas of the country are at greater risk at certain times of the year. Coastal areas are at greater risk for flooding during hurricane season (i.e., June to November), while the Midwest is more at risk in the spring and during heavy summer rains. Ice jams occur in the spring in the Northeast and Northwest. Even the deserts of the Southwest are at risk during the late summer monsoon season.

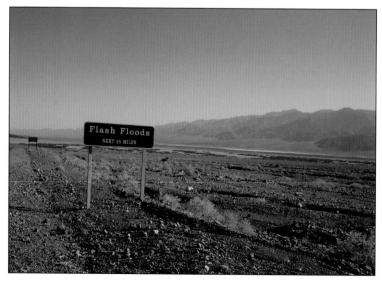

A flash flood warning sign in Death Valley.

Generally, the natural behavior of water (and flowing water) is that it moves from higher ground to lower ground, meaning that it travels the path of least resistance. This means if there is a higher ground adjacent a lower ground, the lower ground is a lot more likely to experience floods. Additionally, anywhere that rains fall, floods can develop. This means that anytime the rains bring more water than can be drained or absorbed by the soil, there is a flood potential.

There are three major flood types: Flash floods; rapid on-set floods and slow onset floods; and one minor one, urban floods.

A flash flood is a sudden transformation of an arroyo or small stream into a violent burst of water usually occurring after heavy rain, broken dam or rapid snowmelt. More severe flash floods can rip out trees, destroy buildings and bridges, scour new channels, and sweep away cars. There is usually no warning, no preparation, and the impact is immediate and devastating. Flash floods are the number one weather-related killer in the US. Nearly half of all flash-flood fatalities are auto related.

Rapid on-set floods are similar to flash floods, but these take longer to develop and the flood can last for a day or two. Rapid onset floods are destructive, but they are not as surprising. With rapid onset floods, people save some property and get out of the way before the flooding gets bad.

Slow on-set floods are usually the result of bodies of water flooding over their banks. These floods tend to develop slowly and can last for days and even weeks. They aren't limited to a river channel and often spread over many miles. They occur mostly in flood plains.

Urban flooding occurs when low-lying impenetrable ground (concrete, asphalt) becomes saturated. Rainfall is unable to run off as quickly as it accumulates. Coastal and estuary flooding is caused by high tidal surges and waves that damage the coast. These unusual tides and surge are caused by tsunamis, hurricanes, or tropical storms.

Causes of flooding:

- Heavy rains that last anywhere from a few hours to a few days saturate the ground so much that water has nowhere to go.

- Waterways—like streams, rivers, and lakes—cannot contain rain and/or snowmelt, resulting in overflow.
- Waterways become blocked with debris or ice, water backs up, and diverts its path, often flooding the nearby banks.
- Water systems break, including levees, dams, sewer, and public water systems.
- Storm surges push seawater onto land, flooding coastal areas, and beyond.

Major American Floods Since 1810

1936 St. Patrick's Day
1955 Hurricanes Connie & Diane
1972 Tropical Storm Agnes
1975 Tropical Storm Eloise
1996 January Basinwide Flash Flood
2004 Tropical Storm Ivan
2005 Katrina
2017 Harvey

One-Hundred-Year Flood

You might have read about a more recent flood being called a one-hundred-year or five-hundred-year flood. You might have thought that a one-hundred-year flood was the level of flood that was so terrible it only occurs once a century. Not exactly. According to insurance language, the one-hundred-year flood is one that has a 1 percent, or one out of one hundred, chance of being equaled or exceeded in any given year. A five-hundred-year flood has even less of a chance of occurring. The term gives an estimate of the probability that a flood of a certain size will occur, not when it will occur. So two one hundred-year floods could occur in the same year . . . and they have recently.

The most common type of flood is a river flood. If the river's capacity is more than its flow rate, then flooding occurs in the surrounding area of the river. An extreme river flood is called a flash flood, which carries water ranging from ten to twenty feet high. This event occurs very fast without warnings or extreme rains. It happens because of a natural or man-made river blockage, such as dams, glaciers, or landslides, releasing an immense volume of water.

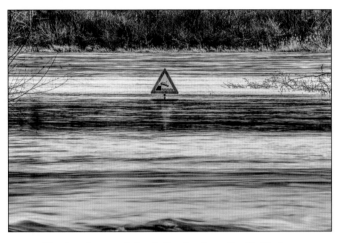

Nearly submerged sign in floodwaters. *Credit: Pixabay.*

Riverine Floods

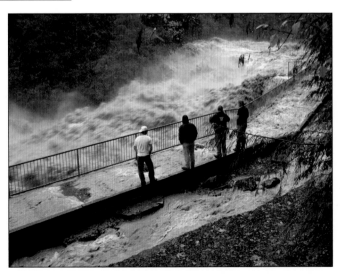

Granite Falls on the Stillaguamish River, Washington at nine feet above flood stage. *Credit: iegmund, CC-BY-SA-3.0 creativecommons. org licenses by-sa 3.0.*

A Flood Warning or Flood Watch generally refers to the flood potential of rivers and major streams. This can result from heavy rainfall or melting snow over a wide area, causing rivers to swell and inundate large areas. Downstream areas may flood well after the rainfall has ended or in areas where no rain occurred.

There are several stages of river floods:

- **Action Stage:** River level is near full, but below flood stage. At some locations there are pre-determined actions that must be taken, such as closing roads or increasing of staff levels for emergency workers.
- **Flood Stage:** The river is overflowing its banks and minor flooding begins in unprotected low-lying areas.
- **Moderate Flood Stage:** Flooding inundates some structures and roads near rivers and streams. Some locations require evacuation of people and/or transfer of property to higher elevations.
- **Major Flood Stage:** Flooding of developed areas results in extensive inundation of structures and roads and requires significant evacuations of people and/or transfer of property to higher elevations.

Flood Facts

- Tropical cyclones, hurricanes, tsunamis, and high tidal waves damage coastal barricades, resulting in coastal flooding.
- Two thirds of flood deaths occur in vehicles. Most cases occur when drivers make the deadly mistake of driving through floodwaters.
- Floods occur everywhere, even in the desert.
- The word "flood" comes from an old English word that means "a flowing of water, river, or sea."

- Ice jam flooding happens when heavy rain causes ice to break into pieces and form a barricade. The water stored behind the barricade builds to mass then spills over into the surrounding area. Eventually, the barricade will break, and that water flows rapidly downstream.

- Rapidly-moving water is dangerous and so powerful it can wash a car, house, tree, or person away. Two feet of flood water can lift and move even large vehicles.

- In recent years, some US states make citizens reimburse the cost of their rescue when they drive into flooded areas.

- Since 1900, floods have taken more than ten thousand lives in the United States.

- The 1976 Big Thompson Flood in Colorado killed 144 people and created almost $40 million worth of damages. Ninety-five percent of those killed in this flash flood tried to beat the waters along their way, instead of climbing rocks or going uphill to higher grounds.

- The 1993 Mississippi River Flood covered a five-hundred-mile long and two-hundred-mile wide area, and destroyed over fifty thousand homes, twelve thousand miles of farmland, and did $20 billion in damages.

- In Ancient Egypt, people relied on the Nile River floods because they created enriched soil for farmers.

Preparation

Need a good reason you should prepare for a flood? Standard homeowner's insurance does not cover floods, so that means if your fancy furniture is ruined, your carpet soiled, your walls so soaked that all need replacing, your homeowner's insurance does not compensate.

Preparation includes buying additional coverage for floods. The number one cause of weather-related deaths in the United States? Flash floods. These can happen anywhere in America, at any time. Tsunamis cause floods. Hurricanes cause floods. Snowmelt, heavy rain, jammed rivers, and broken dams all cause floods. So start preparing.

Flood preparedness goes beyond an emergency kit and evacuation route. First, you should learn the difference in emergency weather announcements so you can know your risk. The National Weather Service is responsible for issuing flooding watches and warnings, which are typically announced on local television channels, public radio, NOAA weather radios, texts, and apps. Be a part of your community flood prevention, too. Communities can work toward flood prevention through coastal defense walls, retaining walls, levees, dams, holding ponds or basins, town planning, bayou or waterway system, drainage improvement, debris removal, adding strategic vegetation, and most especially, educating the public.

Your goal now, before a flood occurs, is to reduce the risk of damage to structures from flooding. This means elevating critical utilities, such as electrical panels, switches, sockets, wiring, appliances, and heating systems, and waterproofing basements. In areas prone to flooding, you should consider elevating the entire structure.

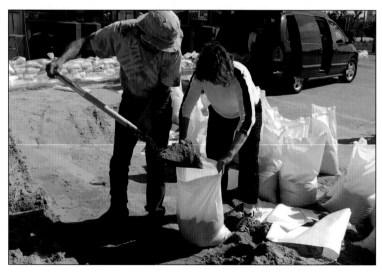

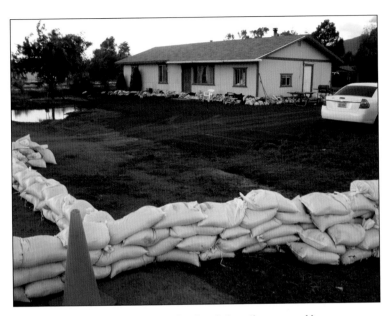

Prepare sandbags before a flood and place them around homes, buildings, and other areas you want to protect. *Credit: Don Becker, USGS; Deborah Lee Soltesz.*

If you live in a frequently-flooded area, think about stockpiling emergency building materials if you have room to store them. These supplies include plywood, plastic sheeting, lumber, nails, hammer and saw, pry bar, sand, shovels, sandbags and a variety of sealable plastic tubs (to store your valuables) and a pair or two of chest waders. You can do a lot around the house to help thwart the effects of flooding. Plant trees and shrubs and lots of vegetation in your yard to control erosion and help slow the speed of floodwater.

Things to do First

- Know your flood risk. Check with local authorities and your insurance agent to know more about flood risk for your home.
- Discover and become a part of your local emergency plans. The plans will include where to go, and how to get there

(typically higher ground), the highest level of buildings, or plans and routes to evacuate.

- Create your own flood emergency plan for local flood risk including evacuation, emergency kits, and shelter destinations with various locations for high ground.
- Create an evacuation plan for your household and build emergency preparedness kits for each in your family, including a minimum of three days of food and water, flashlights, batteries, cash, and first-aid supplies.
- Avoid building in a floodplain. If you do, it's important to elevate and reinforce your home.
- Elevate your furnace, water heater, and electric panel if they are susceptible to flooding.
- Install check valves in sewer traps to prevent flood water from backing up into the drains of your home.
- Construct barriers (levees, beams, floodwalls) to stop flood water from entering.
- Seal walls in basements with waterproofing compounds to avoid seepage.
- Waterproof the basement. Install sump pumps with battery backup in case of a power failure. Installing a water alarm will alert you if water is collecting in your basement.
- Talk to your insurance agent about buying flood insurance. Flood insurance is available for homeowners, renters, and business owners. Because homeowner's insurance policies do not typically cover flood losses, you will need to purchase separate flood insurance if your property is at risk for flooding. Flood insurance takes thirty days to take effect.
- If you live in a high-risk flood zone, flood insurance may be a requirement. To know your home's risk, FEMA has created Flood Insurance Rate Maps, referred to as FIRMs, which details each area's risk for flooding.
- In areas with repetitive flooding, as costly as this might be (consider the costs otherwise) consider elevating the building.

- Keep gutters and downspouts free of debris.
- Complete a household inventory. Take photos or video and write down all the inventory, condition, details, and value.
- Learn how to shut off utilities; your electricity, water, and gas lines. It doesn't hurt to teach others in your household to do this in case you're not home.
- Stay up to date on your family's tetanus shots. If it floods, the chances you cut yourself on underwater obstacles increases.
- If you have young children, be sure to talk to them about the dangers of flood water; many don't realize the force and power behind a flood and attempt to play in the water.

Emergency Kit:

Create an emergency kit for each member of the household, one for the car, and one for work. Your basic kit for a flood should look like this:

- Prescriptions and other medicines you might need.
- First-aid kit (either build your own or make sure to add include bandages, antibacterial creams, antihistamines, syringes, splints, and a suture kit).
- Extra eyeglasses (or cheaters if you need them).
- Power cords for any device you have (including a solar charger in case the power is out).
- Batteries.
- Flashlights (we like to have two smaller intense flashlights and one headlamp in each kit).
- Important papers (birth certificates, insurance papers, passports, contracts, medical papers, bank account numbers, etc.) flash drives, hard drives (all in a zippered bag.) Ideally, you also have all this information backed up safely on the Cloud as well.
- Water for three days (one gallon per day). That's a lot to carry in a backpack so stuff as many water bottles as you can in your kit.

- A water filter (like the backpackers carry) and/or purification tablets to make water potable.
- Radio (with batteries) and a hand-crank radio.
- Food: At least three to five days' worth of non-perishable food estimating at around two thousand calories per day, per person.
- Hygiene items like toothpaste, toothbrush, shampoo, feminine products, deodorant, etc.
- A map of the local area in case you don't have power, you'll need to know how to get around.
- An extra set of car and house keys.
- Shoes. We're fisherman and have used lightweight sandals designed for wading. They are lightweight, have grip, and are ideal for the kit. Flip-flops won't work in flood conditions (they will come off, leaving your feet exposed to underwater dangers), but shoes designed for wading will keep you better protected. A pair of old canvas slip-on tennis shoes with a thick rubber sole would work too.
- Duct tape. You always need duct tape.
- To-do list of things that should be done before you leave if you must evacuate and how to do them.
- Emergency contact list, including names, phone numbers, and addresses.
- Deck of cards in case you have to wait for a long period.
- Pen and notepad in case you have to leave a note or take down information.
- Cash and change. ATMs are likely to be without cash or without power.

Gather and store supplies for all your common locations in case you need to stay in place during a flood. Using trash bags tied up and perhaps even secured at the knot with duct tape will protect your supplies. A good idea is to use Ziploc baggies of all sizes to waterproof all kinds of paperwork and important items.

Family Evacuation Plan

If your local government issues evacuation orders, don't think you need to be brave or stubborn and stick around. You need to evacuate if mandated by local government, which usually has more information about the pending flood than the general public.

While most communities have their own specific evacuation plan, you need to have one just for your family, making sure you have two additional backup plans. You'll want to have multiple options if you encounter flooded roads, fallen trees, downed power lines or any other obstacle that forces you off your planned route.

Choose an out-of-state emergency contact and ensure each person in your household has that person's name, telephone number, and address (preferably in their smartphone.) If a flood occurs and the family is separated, this person is the primary contact so each family member can check in to verify their safety. Communities usually have local relief centers set up in emergencies. Find out where they are ahead of time.

Have each member download the NOAA Weather app on their phone. If wireless services are out during an emergency, there are several messaging apps that also allow phone calls on your cell data, so search those out and install on each phone.

Flash foods often come with no warning whatsoever; in fact, it might not have even rained where you are to experience a flash flood. If you live downhill of heavy rain, or along a stream or ditch, the water that collects from above you can come rushing down with amazing speed and fury.

People can expect a Flood Watch and a Flood Warning announcement if the rain falls one or more inches/hour for over three days in a row. Three alerts that local officials will send out about flooding:

1. **Flood Watch**: A message that flooding is possible and to listen to local radio or TV news and weather for more information.

2. **Flood Warning**: A message that flooding will occur soon, if it hasn't already, and to move to higher ground or evacuate immediately.

3. **Flash Flood**: A flood that can happen within minutes or hours of heavy rainfall, a dam or levee failure, or city drains overflowing.

So when should you perk up and be alert for a flood?

- If it has been raining hard for several hours, or steadily raining for several days, be alert to the possibility of a flood.

- Turn on your NOAA Weather Radio or a portable, battery-powered radio (or television) for updated emergency information; or use your NOAA app. Local stations typically provide the best advice for your particular situation.

- If you are in your vehicle, camp or park away from streams and arroyos (washes), particularly during threatening conditions. Even if it's dry where you are, flash floodwaters rise so quickly, the rushing water can crash through camp and carry you or your belongings away.

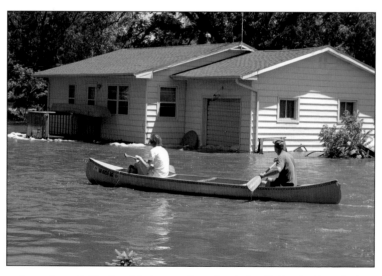

Assessing neighborhood damages after a flood. *Credit: Don Becker, USGS.*

- When in or along stream channels, be aware of distant events, such as dam breaks or thunderstorms that may cause flash floods in the area. Have emergency supplies in place at home, at work, and in the car.

During a flood, listen for updates from the local authorities. You must move important items to a safe place or higher floor of the house. Do not go out and walk through the road where the water is moving. Stay tuned to your phone alerts, TV, or radio for weather updates, emergency instructions, or evacuation orders.

- Check on your neighbors to make sure they're okay.
- Know what to do before, during, and after a flood.
- Listen to local officials via radio, TV, or social media.
- Evacuate when advised by authorities or if you are in a flood or flash flood prone area.

HURRICANE FLOODING

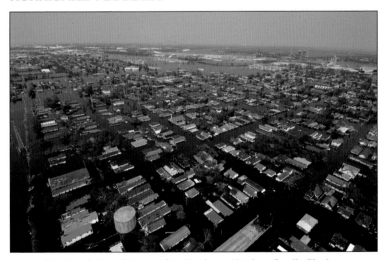

Flooding in New Orleans after Hurricane Katrina. *Credit: Pixabay.*

This is a special type of flooding. You have seen the images of people trapped on top of their house for days. These kinds of epic floods can destroy homes, keep occupants trapped for days and days, cause serious water contamination, and disrupt emergency management services, so if you live where this kind of serious flooding can happen, you need to prepare in a special way.

Your attic needs to have an escape hatch or you need to take a saw or axe up there to be able to make an exit. Take something to make an SOS sign for first responders to see you. Have extra non-perishable food and water in tubs you can store in the attic in case you have to find refuge up there. A couple of pairs of chest waders would come in handy if you have to move about in the floodwater. Round up some life vests from your boat and store them in the garage.

Survival

A flood is imminent. Not going out into a flood is your best bet of survival. You've listened to the flood warning, gotten to higher ground, and you're not out driving yet, so you're likely to survive. But there are things you can do now, before it gets bad, which will increase your safety and the protection of your property.

So it's raining and you think you might have severe flooding, and perhaps you've gotten a flash flood watch and you have time, do these things (but use common sense on timing):

- Put important things in waterproof containers.
- Elevate what you can, including photo albums, important documents, and anything else that can be moved to an upper level of the home, attic or second floor.
- Anchor fuel tanks, boats, and anything else outside that is not securely attached to the ground.
- Move lawn furniture indoors because if it's outside, and the water gets high enough, it will beat against your house.
- If things are dire, you may have to place sandbags around your property to divert water, or at least slow it down.
- If ordered to evacuate, be sure to shut off electric, gas, and water.
- Fill the bathtub, sink, and water bottles with fresh water because your water source could be halted or contaminated.
- Fill up your vehicle's gas tank.

- Have someone stay listening to local TV or radio, or a NOAA radio, for weather updates.
- If your community issues warning sirens, listen up.
- Keep pets safe with you during a potential flood. One of the biggest problems with our recent hurricanes was that dog owners left pets leashed in the backyard. When the floods came, many animals perished. If you can't take your pet, at least give them a chance to survive.
- Move your valuables and furniture to higher levels (attic or second floor.)
- Move hazardous materials (such as paint, oil, pesticides, and cleaning supplies) to higher locations.
- Disconnect electrical appliances. Don't touch these if you they are wet, or if you are wet or standing in water.
- Bring outside possessions indoors or tie them down securely. This includes lawn furniture, garbage cans, and other movable objects.

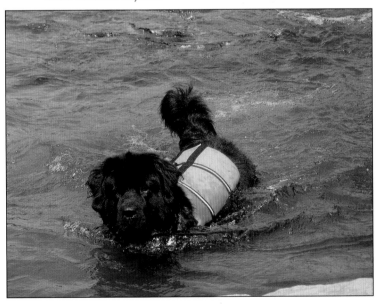

Provide life vests and other protections for your pets during a flood.
Credit: Pixabay.

- Seal any vents to the basement to prevent flooding.
- Make sure everything that is of importance is secured (jewelry, documents, pets, and other valuables) and waterproofed. If you have a second floor, take all the valuables up the stairs.

What to Do During a Flood Watch

- Keep listening to NOAA Weather Radio, or a portable, battery-powered radio (or television) for updated emergency information. Local stations provide you with the best advice for your particular situation. More and more, apps and text alerts are being used.
- Everyone in a watch area should be ready to respond and act immediately. Floods and flash floods can happen quickly and without warning.
- Be alert to signs of flooding, and if you live in a flood-prone area, be ready to evacuate at a moment's notice.
- Follow the instructions and advice of local authorities. Local authorities are the most informed about affected areas. They will best be able to tell you areas to avoid.

Evacuation

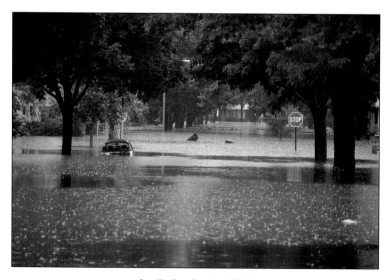

Credit: Don Becker, USGS.

If ordered to evacuate, do so as quickly as possible. Don't ask questions and don't second guess the decision. Grab your emergency kits and go. Quickly disconnect all electrical appliances. If you encounter flooded roads on your evacuation route, turn around and take a different route. Do not drive through water that is more than twelve inches deep.

- Learn your evacuation routes before you ever have to encounter a flood because when you get the evacuation alert, you will be panicky and hurried.
- Prepare for a flood by knowing your evacuation routes, how you will get there, and where you will stay.
- Get your emergency kit bags ready and handy before it ever gets to the evacuation order in case you need to leave quickly due to a flood.
- If the authorities either advise or order an evacuation, do so immediately. Don't dillydally but also make sure you turn off everything, elevate your valuables, and grab your emergency kit bags. As you evacuate, the authorities may not know your exact situation so if the waters are too high to evacuate safely, don't do it.

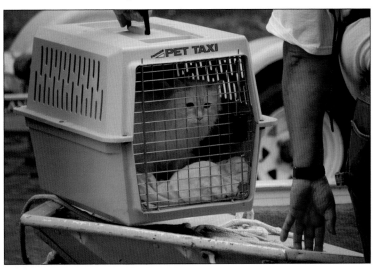

A cat is rescued after a flood. *Credit: Don Becker, USGS.*

- If flooding is imminent or already occurring, evacuate to higher ground if you are in a flood-prone area. But, do not enter floodwaters in order to seek higher ground.

During a flood, water levels and the rate of water-flow change quickly. Get to higher ground. Do not drive or walk into water. It only takes six inches of water to knock you off your feet. Stay informed by monitoring local radio and television for updates. If you're already on "high ground" during a flood, stay where you are. Don't risk your or your family's safety.

Be prepared by having your supplies already stored. Gather the supplies you may need in case a flood leaves you without power, water, or gas.

Walking through flood water is tricky and dangerous. The water may not seem deep or powerful, but that miscalculation has cost many people their lives. What may not seem deep to you might to a shorter person or a child. If the water is six inches and flowing, that's all it takes to knock you off your feet. Any deeper and you could be whisked away.

There may be underwater dangers you can't see—sharp objects, things that might trap your foot or leg, such as a hole, something slippery, or something unstable. The water might be contaminated with bacteria or chemicals. Another real and present danger are downed power lines.

What to Do During a Flood Warning

When a flood or flash flood warning is issued:

- Listen to a NOAA Weather Radio, or a portable, battery-powered radio (or television) for updated emergency information. Local stations provide you with the best advice for your particular situation.
- Be alert to signs of flooding. A warning means a flood is imminent or is happening in the area. Look out your windows and see what is going on around your house.

Disconnect electrical appliances and move valuables to higher areas.

- If you live in a flood-prone area or think you are at risk, evacuate immediately without waiting for an order. Move quickly to higher ground. Save yourself, not your belongings. The most important thing is you and your family's safety.
- Don't forget the pets.

If You're in a Vehicle

The second cause of drowning flood deaths is caused when walking in or near floodwaters; first is drowning while driving your vehicle. Your car should have a full tank of gas. You don't have time or ability to get gas now. Follow recommended routes. Don't sightsee. Avoid disaster areas. Your presence might hamper rescue or other emergency operations and put you at further risk. If for some reason your route has become untenable, your preparation should allow you to quickly choose a new path. In case cell service is out, have a street map of your city.

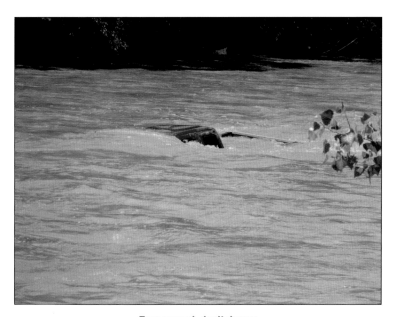

Turn around, don't drown.

Keep an eye out for washed out roads, earth slides, and downed trees or power lines. Nighttime is especially dangerous in floods because it's almost impossible to determine the depth or flow of water. Drive slowly and cautiously. If the vehicle stalls, abandon it. Over half of all flood-related drownings occur when a vehicle is driven into floodwaters.

If you come up on waterflow from the flood, and you can't get a gauge on depth or flow-force, "Turn around, don't drown!" Do not drive around barriers. Do not drive through flooded waters—if it looks like it's tire-high, don't do it. You can lose control of your car in only a few inches of moving water. If your car gets into two feet of more of water, it can float and be swept away. If water rises around your car, leave the vehicle immediately. Climb to higher ground as quickly as possible. Climb up a tree if you believe your life is in danger.

If you happen to be in a vehicle during a flood, remember never to drive through floodwater. It only takes twelve inches of water to pull a compact car away and only two feet of water to sweep away large vehicles. If the water level is rising and you're unable to move the vehicle—or if it stalls and struggles to restart—abandon the car or truck immediately and head toward higher ground. But if the water is too deep and strong, don't risk leaving the vehicle. Instead, stop, call 911, and remain inside (climb onto the roof if water starts to enter your car). If higher ground is not available, find a tall, sturdy object (such as a tree) and climb as high onto it as you can.

<u>If someone falls in or is trapped in flood water:</u>

Do not go after the victim. Use a flotation device. If possible, throw the victim something to help them float, such as a spare tire, large ball, or foam ice chest. Let's be brutally honest: If a loved one goes in, and you jump in after them, the chances are good your family will lose two members instead of one. Call 911. Call for assistance and give the correct location information.

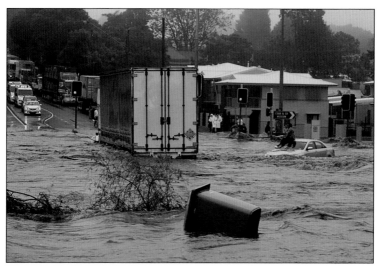

Stranded survivors wait on top of a car after a flood in Toowoomba, Australia.
Credit: Kingbob86 (Timothy), www.flickr.com/photos/kingbob86 5341730273.

Basic Safety Tips

- Turn around, don't drown!
- It's not always possible but when you can, avoid walking or driving through floodwaters.
- Do not drive over bridges that are over fast-moving flood-waters. Floodwaters can scour foundation material from around the footings and make the bridge unstable.
- Just six inches of moving water can knock you down, and one foot of moving water can sweep your vehicle away.
- If there is a chance of flash flooding, move immediately to higher ground.
- If floodwaters rise around your car but the water is not moving, abandon the car and move to higher ground. Do not leave the car and enter moving water.
- Avoid camping or parking along streams, rivers, and creeks during heavy rainfall. These areas can flood quickly and with little warning.

- Avoid already flooded areas and areas subject to sudden flooding. Do not attempt to cross flowing streams. Most flood fatalities are caused by people attempting to drive through water or people playing in high water. The depth of water is not always obvious. The roadbed may be washed out under the water and you could be stranded or trapped. Rapidly rising water may stall the engine, engulf the vehicle and its occupants, and sweep them away. Look out for flooding at highway dips, bridges, and low areas. Two feet of water will carry away most automobiles.
- Do not drive into flooded areas. If floodwaters rise around your car, abandon the car and move to higher ground if you can do so safely. You and the vehicle can be quickly swept away.
- Six inches of water will reach the bottom of most passenger cars, causing loss of control and possible stalling.
- One foot of water will float many vehicles.
- Two feet of rushing water can carry away most vehicles including sport utility vehicles (SUVs) and pickup trucks.
- If you are driving and come upon rapidly rising waters, turn around and find another route. Move to higher ground away from rivers, streams, creeks, and storm drains. If your route is blocked by floodwaters or barricades, find another route. Barricades are put up by local officials to protect people from unsafe roads. Driving around them can be a serious risk.

If you're hoping to stay in your home, or if you cannot evacuate because of high waters, get to the highest floor—but do NOT go into a closed attic. If water levels get too high, you may get trapped inside with no way to exit the building. Take an axe or saw (or both) to the attic so you can get out if needed. If necessary, and only if necessary, climb onto the roof.

Never try to swim to safety; instead wait to be rescued. This has an exception of course—if your house is being swept away or the waters have overtaken the highest point and if you're under imminent threat, you can go. Floodwaters are filled with unseen debris that can hit you, pull you under the water, or even knock you unconscious.

Aftermath

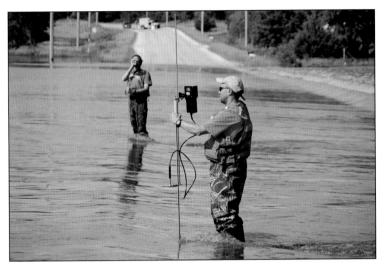

Workers measure after a flood. *Credit: Don Becker, USGS.*

After a flood, the risks still remain. Roads may have weakened or damaged, both standing and moving water will likely be contaminated, and there may be unattended gas leaks and fallen cables. Stay away from contaminated flood water. If your skin comes into contact with contaminated flood water, wash with soap and uncontaminated water as soon as possible. Stay away from moving water. It can knock you off your feet. Stay out of the way of emergency workers so they can do their job easily.

If You Evacuated:

Return home only when authorities say it is safe. Be aware of areas where floodwaters have receded and watch out for debris. Do not attempt to drive through areas that are still flooded. Listen to official public information to get expert, informed advice as soon as it becomes available.

Post Disaster

If you've never been through a flood, you may think that once the water resides, the problems are over. But for many, that's just the beginning. To continue to protect your family and your home, it's important you don't return until local authorities say it's okay and to take some precautions when moving around your neighborhood and home. The impact of the flood on your home and property is affected by a lot variables, including the water level the flood reached, how long the water lingered, how polluted the water was, and how forcefully it flowed.

After a flood, always watch where you walk. Floodwaters are murky so they hide sharp and dangerous debris underwater like broken glass and metal. If there is standing water that you must walk through, but can't see into, use a stick to push through the water in front of you. This alerts you of large debris or unseen risks.

Wear the appropriate protective clothing and gear like boots, gloves, and safety glasses when it comes to moving debris. Flooded homes have

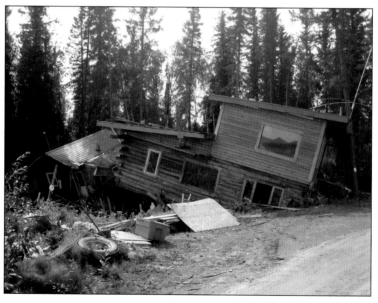

This house moved over three hundred feet after a flood in Alaska.
Credit: Ben Brennan, FEMA Photo Library.

potential hazards. Before you go in, get a professional to check for loose wires, mold, and hidden damage. If you go inside, only use generators or other gas-powered machinery outdoors and away from windows.

Use text messaging or social media to communicate with family and friends and let them know you are okay. Telephones and cellular phone systems are often overwhelmed following a disaster, so use phones only for emergency calls. Texting is better.

When you return home, here are some of the things to be aware of:

- Make sure you have permission from emergency officers to get back inside your house.
- Keep all power and electrical appliances off until the house is cleaned up properly and an electrical personnel has confirmed that it is okay to put them on.
- Make sure you have photographs, videos, or a record of all the damage, as it may be needed for insurance claims.
- Clean the entire home, together with all the objects in it very well before you use them again. They may be contaminated.
- Wear appropriate gear (mask and gloves) before cleaning begins. After a flood, standing water that remains is often polluted with mud, debris, oil, gas, chemicals, and sewer water.
- Floods often cause erosion, which impacts roads, walkways, and bridges; be very careful when working on or around these structures.
- Just as floodwaters erode roads, they also impact the structures and foundations of buildings and homes, making them weak enough to collapse without warning. Check out your foundation.
- Floods increase the possibility of landslides and mudslides, so if you live in an area that's at risk for these disasters, be aware.
- Wild animals often lose their homes during a flood and seek shelter wherever they find it; snakes, especially, are often seen in homes and surrounding areas during and after floods.

Once you're able to return home, the first thing you need to do is assess the damage. Only a few inches of water can cause tens of thousands of dollars in repairs and replacements. Call your flood insurance company immediately to file a claim. And be sure to take pictures of the water level and damage as soon as possible for the insurance company to review. You should have "before" pics of the house and property for comparison and inventory.

Once inside, be aware of the following complications:

- Electrical shock, especially where there is standing water.
- Mold.
- Asbestos.
- Lead paint.
- Loose floorboards.
- Slippery surfaces.
- Gas leaks.
- Wild animals.

When it comes to cleaning up after a flood, here are things you need to do:

- Use a flashlight, never a candle, lantern, or other open flame in case a gas leak is present.
- Throw away any food, even canned items, that have been in contact with floodwaters or been kept at unsafe temperatures due to flooding.
- Check leech beds, septic tanks, or sewer systems for leaks or damage.
- Have your well tested before drinking or cleaning with the water.
- Disinfect every surface that was in contact with flood water; mold and bacteria are possibly everywhere.
- Remove any carpet that got wet during the flood. Rugs can be dried but many will continue to smell fishy.
- Wood and drywall that got saturated with floodwater should be removed and replaced, allowing the framing behind it to completely dry before replacing.

- When dealing with items exposed to floods, such as furniture, clothes, rugs, follow these steps:
  - Air out.
  - Move out.
  - Tear out.
  - Clean out.
  - Dry out.
- Do not turn on electricity until it's been verified safe by an electrician.
- While working in the flooded area, you are surely wearing your protective gear, and you might include wearing a facemask.

Ten Interesting Flood Facts

1. Since 1900, floods have killed ten thousand people in the United States alone.
2. Flash floods often carry water as high as ten to twenty feet.
3. Ninety-five percent of those who perished in the flood tried to outrun the waters along their path rather than climbing rocks or going to a place higher up the ranks.
4. Sixty-six percent of deaths caused by floods usually occur in a vehicle, and most happen when drivers make a single fatal mistake trying to navigate through floodwaters.
5. Just six inches of rapidly moving flood water can make a person fall down.
6. Floods with a height of two feet of water can float a large vehicle, even a bus.
7. A third of roads and bridges are usually destroyed by a flood, and only 50 percent of people will survive when crossing the bridge is destroyed.

(Continued)

8. The Mississippi River Flood of 1993 covered an area five hundred miles long and two hundred miles wide. More than fifty thousand homes were destroyed, and twelve thousand miles of farmland damaged.

9. Hurricanes, winter storms, and snow melt (often overlooked) are the main causes of flooding.

10. The new land development can increase flood risk, especially if the construction changes natural runoff paths.

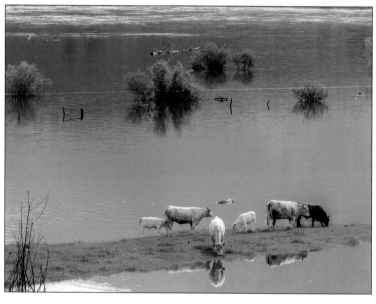

Cows grazing on a small space of unsubmerged grass after a flood.
Credit: Pixabay.

Facts and Tidbits

- No region is safe from flooding. All fifty states are subject to flooding, especially flash floods.
- Flash floods can bring walls of water from ten to twenty feet high. If you've ever seen video of a flash flood in a dry

stream bed, you'll be amazed how tall the rushing water is, how much debris it carries, and what great force it contains.

- A car can be swept away in as little as two feet of water.
- To stay safe during a flood, go to the highest ground of floor possible.
- Floods are the most widespread natural disaster aside from wildfires. Ninety percent of all US natural disasters declared by the president involve some sort of flooding.
- Based on estimates provided by Floodsmart Insurance, a two-thousand-square-foot home undergoing twelve inches of water damage could cost more than $50,000.
- Since flood damage is almost never covered by homeowners insurance, flood insurance is important for people living in high-risk flood zones.

CHAPTER NINE
EARTHQUAKES

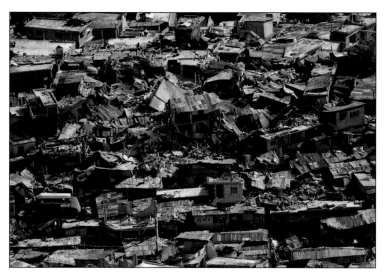

Destruction after a Haitian earthquake.
Credit: legalcode, creativecommons.org licenses 2.0 legalcode.

If you've ever been in an earthquake, then you know it's an intense memory you won't forget. The suddenness, the disorientation, the natural instinct to stay put instead of flee. In an earthquake, you'll often experience violent shaking and sometimes a fluid rolling sensation but always you'll be numbed and overwhelmed with the noise and tumult of things falling. And earthquakes shake more than just our homes or buildings; they also shake our psyches. Earthquakes occur when one of Earth's plates scrapes, bumps, or drags along another plate. When does this happen? Constantly. About a half-million quakes rock the Earth every day. That's millions a year. People don't feel most of them because the quake is too small, too far below the surface, or too deep in the sea. Some, however, are so powerful they can be felt thousands of miles away.

A powerful earthquake can cause landslides, tsunamis, flooding, and other catastrophic events. Most damage and deaths occur in populated areas because the shaking can cause windows to break, structures to collapse, fires to start, and other dangers to happen.

Most of the world's earthquakes occur in the twenty-five-thousand-mile horseshoe-shaped zone known as the Pacific Ring of Fire, which for the most part bounds the Pacific Plate. Massive earthquakes tend to occur along other plate boundaries, too, such as along the Himalayan Mountains. Earthquakes occur throughout the world all day. Most are minor and occur in common earthquake locales like California, Alaska, Mexico, New Zealand, Italy, Nepal, and Japan, but earthquakes can occur almost anywhere—Texas, New York, and even England. Around

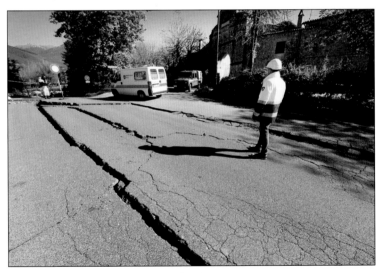

Credit: Pixabay.

500,000 earthquakes occur each year around the world but only about twenty thousand of these can be felt. Only one hundred or so of these earthquakes will do significant damage.

Scientists believe that in the near future, the Pacific Northwest will be hit by a big one, a major earthquake that because of the intersection of great population (seven million people) and the earthquake severity (expected magnitude in the neighborhood of 9.0), will be devastating. Other heavily-populated areas around the world have a history of earthquakes, and when the next one hits, in Japan or Turkey for instance, the results will be devastating.

So what is an earthquake? An earthquake occurs when two blocks of earth suddenly slip past each other. Take a trip back to science class. Perhaps you remember that our earth has four layers: crust, mantle, outer core, and inner core. Just below the surface are tectonic plates and these plates meet other movable plates, called faults. When the plates meet up, stress and friction build energy. When the plates slip and force overcomes friction, that energy is released. The resulting action, the shaking of the earth's surface, is the earthquake (a.k.a. quake, tremor, or temblor). Some earthquakes produce foreshocks, or smaller quakes that occur before the bigger one. The largest earthquake of a sequence is the mainshock. After the mainshock are the aftershocks, the smaller (although sometimes still powerful and often destructive) tremors that follow. These can continue for an indefinite period of time.

You cannot always feel earthquakes. Not all are detectable by human senses. Some earthquakes are so weak that you need a scientist to tell you that you were in it. Others are so strong that countries are violently disrupted and cities thrashed and shaken.

When you think of where most earthquakes occur in America, you naturally think of California. That's a fair assumption. But it's wrong. So what was the state that had the most earthquakes in the lower forty-eight over the last few years? How about the Sooner State? Yes, Oklahoma. Oklahoma experienced 623 magnitude 3.0-plus earthquakes in 2016, 903 in 2015, 579 in 2014, and 109 in 2013. Until 2008, Oklahoma experienced an average of one to two earthquakes of 3.0 magnitude or greater each year, making it by far the most seismically active state in the lower forty-eight.

Each year southern California has about ten thousand earthquakes. Most of them are so small that they are not felt. Only several hundred are greater than magnitude 3.0, and only about fifteen to twenty are greater than magnitude 4.0. Earthquakes of a magnitude of 3.0 earthquakes tend to be felt, while smaller earthquakes may be noticed only by scientific equipment or by people close to the epicenter. We can say with virtual certainty that the increased seismicity in Oklahoma has to do with recent changes in the way that oil and gas are being produced (fracking).

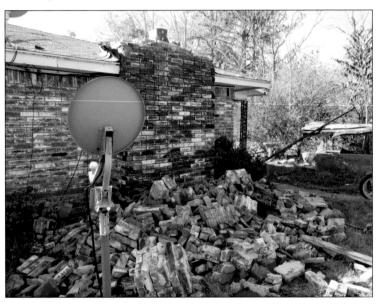

Earthquake damage in Oklahoma. *Credit: Brian Sherrod, USGS.*

If earthquakes can happen in Oklahoma, they can happen anywhere, including where you live or vacation. You think it'll never happen to you but one day, you may find yourself vacationing in San Francisco or Hawaii or Anchorage or Tokyo and you'll be smack in the middle of earthquake territory. We've even experienced earthquakes in the flat plains of Texas.

What is an epicenter? Earthquake ruptures usually begin far under the surface of the Earth. The point of origin miles down is called the hypocenter. The epicenter is the point on the surface directly above the hypocenter. We all grew up hearing about the Richter scale for measuring earthquakes. But since it's an absolute scale, it is an imprecise measurement for scientists. To fully understand things like how the earthquake affected those where the earthquake took place, scientists needed something more. The Modified Mercalli intensity scale does that and gives more precise measurements so as to better distinguish between small, medium and large earthquakes.

There are several ways to measure an earthquake, but the most common is by magnitude. Geologists rate earthquakes in magnitude. Magnitude is the amount of energy released during an earthquake. Scientists no longer use the original Richter scale, but use an updated version. Earthquakes should be referred to as "magnitude X" rather than "an X on the Richter scale." A magnitude 6.0 earthquake releases thirty-two times more energy than a magnitude 5.0 and nearly a thousand times more energy than a 4.0. But that doesn't mean the ground shakes a thousand times harder in a 6.0 than a 4.0, because the energy is released over a much larger area.

The Richter scale is an absolute scale so wherever an earthquake gets recorded, it will measure the same on the Richter scale. The Modified Mercalli differs because it also measures how people feel and react to the shaking of an earthquake.

There are three major factors that influence what you feel in an earthquake: magnitude, your distance from the fault, and local soil conditions. While earthquakes are caused mostly by geological fault adjustment, earthquakes are also caused by other events such as volcanic activity, landslides, mine blasts, and nuclear tests. And earthquakes can cause disasters including tsunamis, floods, fires, soil liquefaction, avalanches and landslides, and . . . building destruction.

Most earthquakes happen fifty miles or less below the Earth's surface. They can happen as deep as 400 miles below the surface. The effects of earthquakes include shaking and ground rupture (remember the Fukushima Nuclear Disaster), volcanic activity, coastal wave attack, wildfires, slope instability leading to landslides and avalanches, soil liquefaction, tsunamis, and floods from damaged dams. The horrific results of an undersea earthquake December 26, 2004 in the Indian Ocean initiated a series of devastating tsunamis. The tsunamis hit the coasts of most all the landmasses bordering the Indian Ocean, killing over a quarter million people in eleven countries.

It's difficult to figure out when an earthquake will occur because the forces that cause plate slippage happen over a large area and over a long period of time but result in forces that affect such a narrow region. We have also gotten better at reducing earthquake risks and saving lives in most at-risk locations, including Mexico. Mexico sits on top of three tectonic plates, so it's one of the most seismically active areas in the world. The Mexican capital, Mexico City, is built on the site of the ancient Aztec city of Tenochtitlan, an island in the middle of a lake. The dry lakebed the city was built upon amplifies shaking from earthquakes. The biggest factor in preventing deaths from earthquakes is employing proper earthquake-resistant building codes. We can design buildings that can withstand most any earthquake, but that is expensive and political.

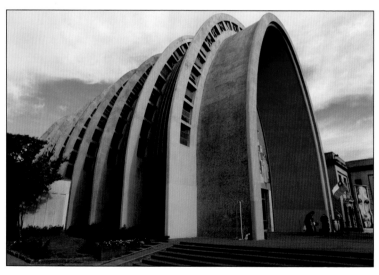

Earthquake resistant cathedral in Chile. *Credit: Walter Mooney, USGS.*

Eliminating certain kinds of buildings, such as flat slab construction, greatly reduces life loss as well, such as flat slab construction. But Mexico has undergone significant changes to building codes and improvements including a much more precise warning system.

The difference in loss of life and property from the big 1985 earthquake in Mexico City to the most recent one in 2017, showed that the improvements worked; fewer lives were lost and more property survived. But in other countries, like Turkey and Iran, they have not made as many improvements and when they get hit by earthquakes, their earthquake resilience isn't up to par and buildings collapse and lives are lost.

Humans can cause or trigger earthquakes as well, too. Filling dams with water, rapidly drawing water from underground reservoirs, underground nuclear testing, fracking, and enhanced geothermal-energy projects all cause so called "induced earthquakes." As an example, due to fracking in Oklahoma, the number of earthquakes surged from a handful a year to 2,500 in 2014, 4,000 in 2015, and 2,500 in 2016.

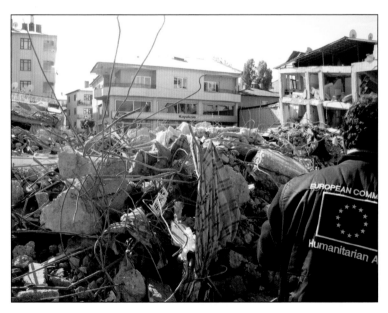

Earthquake damage in Turkey. *Credit: European Commission, DG ECHO.*

One of the first questions that seismologists often get about an earthquake is whether it was a new quake or an aftershock. Most people think that an aftershock is a significantly less dangerous event. But an aftershock of a certain magnitude is no different from an independent temblor of a similar magnitude. The shaking and rupture are the same and the energy released is the same. Aftershocks can actually be more damaging than the initial mainshocks because buildings are already damaged, especially in high population centers.

Preparation

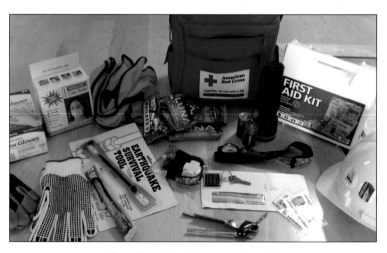

Sample earthquake preparation kit.
Credit: Global X reativecommons.org/licenses/by/2.0/

The keys to preparing for earthquakes occur prior to the event and include: better building codes, earthquake engineering, exterior and interior modification, education, creating a plan, practicing the plan, managing supplies, creating the ideal emergency kit, and readiness combined with awareness.

Building Codes and Earthquake Engineering

So much of true preparation for an earthquake comes in the form of improving building structures to follow earthquake code. This will ensure that both new and older buildings have a good chance of with-standing an earthquake. Nearly two-thirds of the buildings that fell in the 2017 Mexico City earthquake were designed with a flat-slab construction method where the floors are supported only by concrete columns. Flat slabs are now forbidden in parts of the United States, Chile, and New Zealand. In an earthquake, buildings need reinforced walls or lateral bracing and existing buildings can be modified with seismic retrofitting so as to better withstand earthquake forces.

You can't prevent earthquakes but you can improve your home to reduce destructive impact but if you live in an earthquake-risk zone, you really need to bring in a professional to assess your potential hazards and to bring your home to seismic building standards. Ask your pro about home repair, about tips to strengthen your exterior features, such as porches, decks, sliding glass doors, canopies, carports, and garage doors.

Home Modification

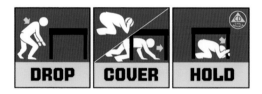

You will want to modify your placement of objects in your home to minimize risk of damage to person and property. In an earthquake, gravity works and things fall. And it's not the shaking that kills you, it's the things that fall on your head. With that in mind, everything from your furniture to home decor will be weaponized if an earthquake hits your home. When the earthquake hits, anything not strapped down or attached to the wall will come crashing down. If you are below, you'll be injured. Make sure your home is securely anchored to its foundation. Strengthen exterior features of the home such as porches, decks, sliding glass doors, canopies, carports, and garage doors. Discuss earthquake insurance with your agent. Depending on your financial situation and the value of your home, it may be worthwhile.

The idea of home modification is to first find safe spaces that you and your family can go to if an earthquake hits. Identify safe places where the furniture is either sturdy or is fastened to the wall, or locate an interior wall in your home. When the shaking starts, follow protocol: Drop, Cover, Hold On. Drop to the ground, Cover your head and neck with your arms, and if a safer place is nearby, crawl to it and Hold On.

Strap down your water heater. During an earthquake, a water heater is basically a missile in your basement. Locate large and heavy objects, find your breakable objects (bottled foods, glass, or china) and place them on lower shelves. If you have cabinets where you store glassware, at least secure the doors where they won't open and spill out the contents. Anchor any overhead lighting fixtures to joists. Anchor top-heavy, free-standing furniture (bookcases, china, and cabinets) to wall studs to keep these from toppling over.

Visualize yourself in your home during an earthquake. Look for things that could easily fall and cause injury. Heavy mirrors, pictures and paintings above beds, big-screen televisions above couches or above

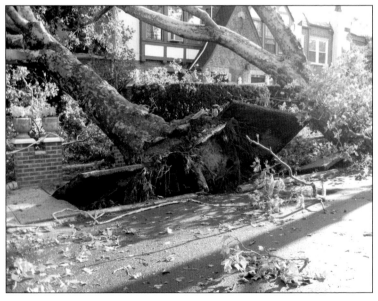

Earthquake uproots trees and uplifts pavement. *Credit: Pixabay.*

your sitting area? Bad move. A bar with lots of big glass bottles of whiskey and vodka, scotch glasses, and decanters? Weapons of glass destruction.

In the basement or garage, make sure your flammable liquids stored away from potential ignition sources such as water heaters, stoves, and furnaces. Learn where the main turn-offs are for your water, gas, and electricity but also teach the others in your household in case you're not home or are incapacitated. Earthquakes can sever a house's pipes and/ or damage electrical lines, creating situations that can easily become deadly. Many use flexible lines for their utilities to avoid breakage.

Planning

Make a plan with your family. No matter when it strikes, you'll want a plan in place. We typically imagine an earthquake occurring while we are at home but what if it happens during school and business hours? Planning ahead of time will help all your loved ones have a better chance at survival. If it's an earthquake with ample power and a killer epicenter, it could leave thousands of people separated from their loved ones with telecommunications systems hampered or shut down, so that it becomes difficult or impossible to track one another down via phone calls, emails, or texts. Ask a friend or relative outside the region to agree to serve as a contact person for your family; if it does become possible to send messages in some form, you're more likely to get through to someone when their end of the communications systems is functional and the lines aren't overloaded.

Plan how you will communicate with family members, including multiple methods by making a family emergency communication plan. Have a survival plan for your home. You and anyone you live with should have a plan to quickly get to safety at a moment's notice. Every member of the house should know exactly what to do and where to go when an earthquake hits. They should know the safe spots in your house—under sturdy tables and against interior walls, especially in corners. They should also know the danger spots in the house—near windows and hanging objects, under big mirrors or paintings. Do you have an evacuation plan with backup routes? Have you remained informed about your community's risk and response plans?

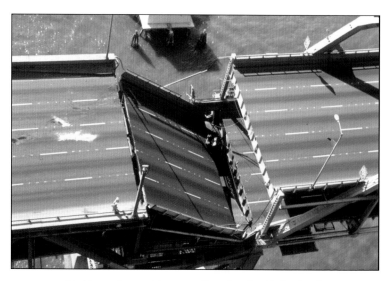

A bridge collapse after an earthquake. *Credit: Joe Lewis.*

Choose a meeting place for your family, remembering that many roads might not be open and that some bridges will be down. Choose a secondary and tertiary meeting spot as well. Find out if your city has designated earthquake gathering areas, where food, water, and first aid will be available. If you have children, learn the earthquake plan at their schools, day-care centers, camps, and after-school activities. Locate your nearest fire and police stations and emergency medical facility. Get to know your neighbors. In most disasters, neighbors become the de-facto first responders, since they are already on the scene when calamity strikes. Make sure you have access to NOAA radio broadcasts. Find an online NOAA radio station.

- Conduct practice drills every six months or so to ensure you and your loved ones know exactly what to do in the event of an earthquake.
- Download an emergency app for iPhone or Android.
- Decide beforehand how and where your family will reunite if separated during a quake and to conduct in-home practice drills. That's the only way to ensure that everyone is on the same page.

- Teach all members of your family about earthquake safety. This includes:
  - The actions you should take when an earthquake occurs.
  - The safe places in a room such as under a strong desk or along interior walls.
  - The danger areas, places to avoid such as near windows, large mirrors, hanging objects, heavy furniture, and fireplaces.
- Learn first aid and CPR. If one of your family members is hurt in an earthquake, basic knowledge of first aid will be a lifesaver. Take a basic first-aid course and become CPR-certified so that if the worst happens, you'll be ready to save lives.
- Find out which of your neighbors has an elderly relative on a ventilator, which one has a generator, which one has a past as a paramedic. Knowing facts like these about each other can save lives: theirs or yours.

Emergency Supplies

Put together your emergency supplies. Keep a flashlight and any low-heeled shoes by each person's bed. Once the shaking begins, you won't have time or sense to locate either. You'll want enough supplies for yourself and your entire family. You'll want enough to last several days or a week. Why a week? You just don't know how bad the earthquake will be or when help will arrive. You may lose electricity or water. You may have access to rescue cut off for a while.

We recommend having the supplies in several locations, including a backpack for each member and a storage container to keep out water or debris. This way you have supplies at your house in case you get stuck there and you have transportable supplies in your backpacks in case you need to leave.

Let's start with stockpiling your supplies for your house. Fresh water is your most important supply. Buy several big packages of individual bottles of water. Store them in the basement or garage. Your earthquake disaster kit should be stored in a durable container such as two thirty-gallon open head drums (which include a bolt-on lid) since not much is likely to damage a steel drum; this means any food, emergency water, and emergency electronics stored inside are likely to make it through a major earthquake intact. Wrap up anything breakable or electronic in your blankets or coats. Not everyone has space to store big drums. You can store smaller amounts in plastic tubs or containers in closets or perhaps an outdoors shed. If you are left without electricity, in the short term, you need flashlights and portable lights. Longer, you'll need a generator. Hand-cranked lights are great additions to your storage in case batteries go out.

Acquire and store non-perishable foods. Make sure to have lots of protein. You might consider backpack survival foods. Peanut butter crackers, powdered soups, and granola bars are ideal. Store at least a three-day supply of non-perishable food. It's best to have enough canned and dried foods sufficient for a week for each member of your household. Note: both water and food stores should be replaced every

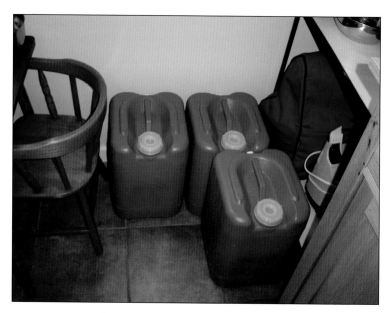

Prepare by filling and storing water jugs.
Credit: John Markos O'Neill, creativecommons.org/licenses/by-sa/2.0/.

so often to maintain freshness. Canned goods have a normal shelf-life of one year for maximum freshness.

Check your supplies every so often. Did a mouse get in? Did anything go bad? Are your batteries fresh? You need a gallon of water per day per person, enough for three days. If you can store more, for a week, do so. Also, pack purification tablets or chlorine bleach (sixteen drops per gallon of water) to purify water if you have to get it from other sources.

Other things you need to complete your earthquake emergency kits:

- First-aid kit. Don't just buy your garden-variety first-aid kit from the discount store. Buy a nice one and even still, add your own flair for your own needs.
- Money, since ATMs may not be operating.
- Simple clothing for all four seasons. But you'll want to be warm no matter what so make sure to include a jacket for each and a change of shoes and socks.
- Blankets, preferably the packaged space-age silvery folded blankets but it makes sense to include one or two normal blankets.
- Surgical masks to protect against dust kicked up from the quake.
- Fire extinguisher that is suitable for all types of fires.
- Portable radio: we suggest battery-operated radio and a hand-cranked radio. We suggest a NOAA radio.
- Extra batteries for all your electronics.
- Medication that is in date, safe from moisture, and enough for a week's time or longer.
- Tools, including a basic tool box and an adjustable or pipe wrench to turn off gas or water, as well as utility knife.
- Baby and pet food if you have either.
- Alternate cooking source like a small charcoal or propane grill or camp stove. You may want to boil water if you have to get it from a source you don't trust. Use of such stoves should not take place until it is determined that there is no gas leak in the area. Also, charcoal should only be burned

outdoors; use of charcoal indoors will lead to carbon monoxide poisoning.

- Bic lighters and wooden matches in a waterproof container.
- Emergency fire starter; essentially anything from an emergency candle to dried tinder in a waterproof container to
  dryer lint or cotton balls that have been dabbed in Vaseline.
  There are several emergency fire starters to choose from;
  having more than one helps ensure you can get a fire going
  with no problem.
- Non-electric, hand-held can opener. Also, a bottle opener
  and non-breakable eating and drinking utensils.
- Waterproof, heavy-duty plastic bags.
- Shovel.
- Toilet paper. It's wise to store more than you think you
  need. Add hand wipes in case you don't have water.
- Disinfectant and hand sanitizer. Sewer lines may have been
  disrupted during the earthquake. Remember that thirty-
  gallon steel drum mentioned above? That drum can double
  as emergency waste storage for any human waste. But you
  will have a buildup of methane gas so put the waste in plastic bags.
- Nylon rope or military spec, paracord, and duct tape.
- Portable fire escape ladder for homes/apartments with
  multiple floors.
- Telephone numbers of police, fire, and doctor. Also, make
  sure you have access to a phone.
- Copies of important papers should be kept in a fireproof
  container or a safe deposit box with a key you always carry.
- Spare eyeglasses and contacts, as well as contact solution.

If the disaster's bad enough and you can't get to your house or your
house is damaged, all the hotels will be full. That means your car's back-
seat becomes your bedroom. Pack protective clothing, rainwear, and
bedding or sleeping bags in your kit, as well as extra blankets and heavy
clothing, including rubber-soled shoes and work gloves.

Packed emergency kits are a necessity, since a quake can leave you homeless in a matter of minutes. Have them stored right by the exit door to your home, perhaps one in your vehicle. You might not have time to track them down. You'll still have your big storage drum in the garage.

Keep a spare set of keys by your bed, in case your other set is inaccessible or can't be found due to the craziness of an earthquake.

Make a lanyard that holds a simple photo ID, including your address and phone number, for each member of the family. Put them on in case of emergency. For very young children, buy a set of safety tattoos that you can quickly apply to an arm or a leg to help ID an injured or lost kid. Dog tags are a must too.

Survival

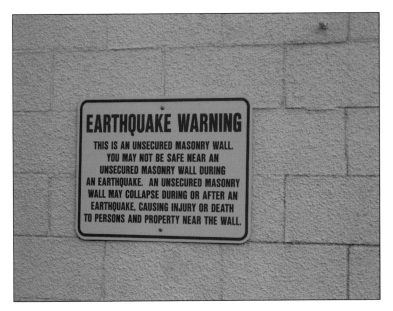

Credit: David Weekly, creativecommons.org.licenses.by.2.0.

It's not the shaking that hurts you. It's the stuff that falls on your head. Collapsing walls, flying glass, and falling objects cause most quake-related injuries and deaths. Stay clear of windows, fireplaces, or appliances if a quake hits. Get under a desk or table, or hold on to a desk or table, or stand against an interior wall. You don't want to be near exterior walls, glass, heavy furniture, fireplaces, and appliances. The kitchen is a particularly dangerous spot what with knives, blenders, coffee pots, and appliances tied into water, electrical, and gas. If you're in an office building, stay away from windows and outside walls and do not use the elevator. The American Red Cross suggests using the drop, cover, and hold method. Drop, cover your eyes by pressing your face against your arm, and hold on. Teach children this method as well.

So the earthquake has just started and you are in the house. Drop down onto your hands and knees so the earthquake doesn't knock you down because if it's big enough, it will. Cover your head and neck with your arms to protect yourself from falling debris. If you sense you are in danger from falling objects, and you determine you can move safely, don't stand and instead crawl for additional cover under a sturdy desk or table or against an interior wall.

Stay away from glass, windows, outside doors, and walls. Move as little as possible. Most injuries occur when folks are moving around, thus falling and injuring themselves with sprains, fractures, and head injuries. If you are in bed, stay there, curl up, hold on, and cover your head.

If you are in the kitchen, you want to get out. Turn off the stove or oven if you are cooking. If you can turn off the gas before you get out, do so. But get out of the kitchen.

Stay where you are until the shaking stops. Do not run outside. Do not get in a doorway as this does not provide protection from falling or flying objects, and you may not be able to remain standing.

If you're in a crowded public place, don't panic. Don't rush for the exits. Get low, stay low, cover your head and neck with your hands and arms, and wait for the shaking to stop. Use stairs and not the elevator. Be aware you may hear loud alarms and you may get wet because smoke alarms and sprinkler systems often go off in buildings because of an earthquake. If you smell gas, get out of the building or your house immediately, and move as far away as possible. Before you leave any

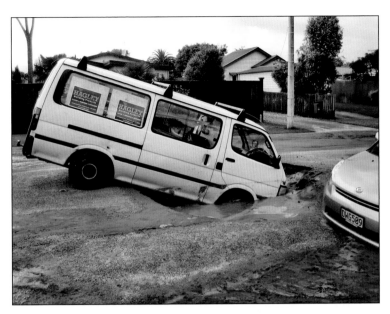

Cars in a sinkhole after an earthquake. *Credit: Martin Luff, creativecommons. org/licenses/by-sa/2.0/legalcode.*

building, look up, and check to make sure that there is no debris from the building that could possibly fall on you.

If you're outside, get into the open. Be observant of sinkholes, faults, and falling debris. Stay clear of buildings because parts of that structure may be falling; avoid power lines, street lights, big signs, or anything else that could fall on you. Find a clear spot and drop to the ground. Stay there until the shaking stops. If you are in a mountainous area watch out for falling rock, landslides, trees, and other debris that could be loosened by quakes. Wait a little bit before you move to another place because aftershocks could immediately follow right after the earthquake.

If you are driving, quickly but carefully move your car as far out of traffic as possible and stop. Do not stop on or under a bridge or overpass or under trees, but pull over to a clear location and come to a complete stop. Listen to local radio to stay informed of the latest traffic and earthquake information. You may have passengers so you need to stay calm so they will too. Avoid bridges and overpasses. Stay inside with your seatbelt fastened until the shaking stops. If a power line falls on your

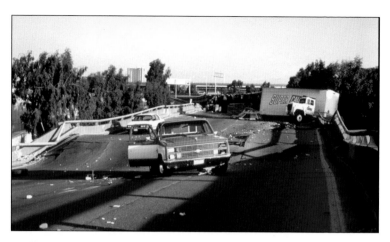

Upper deck of the Nimitz Freeway in California after a devastating 1989 earthquake. *Credit: Joe Lewis.*

vehicle, do not get out. Call 911 and wait for assistance. If you are in a parking garage, treat it as though you are in a building. Get out of your car and get low, and if you can, find an interior wall to crouch beside. A garage is a risky place because of the potential for falling concrete.

After the quake, you're first instinct will be to go home but until you know traffic and other conditions, do not try to rush back to your home. Drive observationally and carefully, avoiding bridges and ramps that may have been damaged looking for breaks in the pavement, as well as sinkholes, fallen rocks, bumps in the road swollen bridge, ramp approaches or any other new hazards.

No matter if you are inside, outside, or in your vehicle, do not expect firefighters, police, or paramedics to be there immediately for you. They may not be available and may be taking care of a big emergency situation. You do want to alert them to your position and condition but your safety in the minutes and perhaps hours after the earthquake are up to you.

Aftermath

Aftershocks are likely and possible at any time. They can collapse weakened buildings, bridges, and other structures. Aftershocks can range

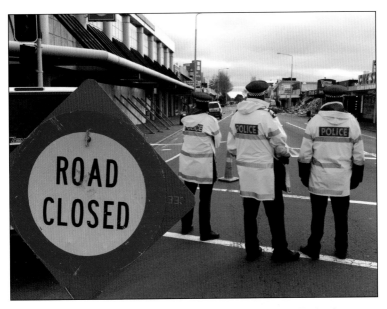

The aftermath of an earthquake in Christchurch, New Zealand.
Credit: Greg O'Beirne, creativecommons.org.licenses.by.2.0.

from imperceptible to equal the power of the original quake itself. Each time you feel an aftershock, drop, cover, and hold on. Aftershocks occur minutes, days, weeks, and even months following an earthquake.

Check yourself for injuries and get first aid, if necessary, before helping injured or trapped persons. Avoid roads, bridges, or ramps that might have been damaged by the earthquake. Don't do anything crazy. Wait for city, municipal, state, or national relief efforts. Look for alerts on your phone and listen to the radio.

When the shaking stops, look around. If you see a clear path to safety, exit the building and find an open space away from danger. If you are at home and the earthquake has passed—time to get ready and get to work. Put on long pants, a long-sleeved shirt, sturdy shoes, and work gloves to protect against injury from broken objects. Look quickly throughout the home and outside of it for damage. If you discover problems, get everyone out.

If you smell or hear a gas leak, get everyone outside and open windows and doors. If you can do it safely, turn off the gas at the meter. Report the leak to the gas company and fire department. Do not use any electrical appliances because a tiny spark could ignite the gas. Don't light a match or a lighter.

If the power is out, unplug major appliances to prevent possible damage when the power is turned back on. If you see sparks, frayed wires, or smell hot insulation, turn off electricity at the main fuse box or breaker. If you will have to step in water to turn off the electricity, you should call a professional to turn it off for you.

Once you've got everyone safe, monitor the local news reports through radio, TV, social media, and cell phone text alerts for emergency information and instructions. Be prepared to drop, cover, and hold on in the likely event of aftershocks.

Stay clear of windows, fireplaces, or heavy appliances in case of aftershocks. Listen to local officials, stay off your phone unless it's an emergency, and don't drive unless absolutely necessary. Learn about the emergency plans that have been established in your area by your state and local government. In any emergency, always listen to the

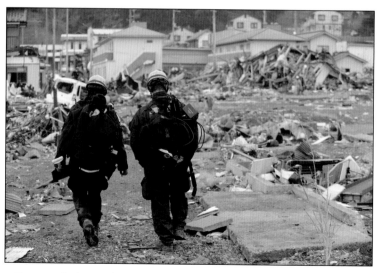

Recovery in Japan after an earthquake. *Credit: Tech. Sgt. Daniel St. Pierre, creativecommons.org/licenses/by/2.0/.*

instructions given by local emergency management officials who know the up-to-the-minute dangers. You and your family might have to go to an earthquake-safe location previously designated by local officials, such as a nearby park. Stay calm, stay aware, and government help should be on the way soon.

You might be buried and unable to move. If you are trapped, don't panic. Save your energy and conserve your oxygen. Tap on something, anything, where people could learn your position, especially metal. Save your voice until you hear someone for certain. Listen, conserve, tap, and listen. There are countless stories from earthquakes around the world where people were rescued days after the fact, which means that your perseverance, your calmness, and your will are all important. Teach your kids to tap on anything if they are ever trapped underneath furniture or other debris. Unfortunately, the longer you are trapped, every hour that goes by the chances of survival decrease significantly.

All too often, the earthquake rubble that traps a person becomes one's tomb. So what are the major factors for survival for a person held hostage by earthquake debris?

- Injuries: Head trauma, broken bones, and damaged organs are the main injuries that will lead to a quicker death. Lesser injuries that are manageable, ones that don't lead to bleeding or internal disturbance, allow survivors to last longer.
- Food and water: If you have access to food and water, your injuries are minor, and you have enough oxygen, you could survive for quite a while. Water is more important than food. Metabolism also plays a part, as does the extra fat you have stored.
- Oxygen: You have to breathe to live.
- Crush syndrome: Injured bodies suffer initially from a buildup of toxins, which causes renal damage. The toxins from the shock can cause the body to be overwhelmed and renal failure can occur. Over time, the tissue will also degrade.
- Other factors include ambient temperature, carbon dioxide levels, loss of fluids, your overall health, and your age.
- Willpower.

If you are trapped but aren't buried, and you have a working cell phone with you, use it to call or text for help. Be pragmatic about using it in order to preserve its battery. Be alert for signs of other trapped victims, and listen closely too. Look for and extinguish any fires, a common effect of earthquakes.

Clean up dangerous spills, as gasoline can be fatal if it explodes or ignites. If you only have paper towels, use several layers of them because gasoline is harmful and is very difficult to wash off. Covering gasoline spills with some shovelfuls of sand is a good idea, as well.

Do not drink water from the sink since it may be contaminated. Sewage systems will be damaged in major earthquakes, so do not flush the toilet. Instead, shut off the water system from the main valve. Make sure that you plug up drains from sinks and bathtubs to prevent any sewage backflow.

Inspect the chimney for any damage before using your fireplace. Chimneys are especially vulnerable to damage from earthquakes and if you light a fire and the chimney has damage, that damage could lead to fire.

If you do nothing else: if you are away from home, return only when authorities say it is safe to do so. Check yourself for injuries and get first aid, if necessary, before helping injured or trapped persons. Expect and prepare for potential aftershocks, landslides, or even a tsunami if you live on a coast. Each time you feel an aftershock, drop, cover, and hold on. Aftershocks frequently occur minutes, days, weeks, and even months following an earthquake. Look for and extinguish small fires. Fire is the most common hazard after an earthquake.

- Be careful when driving after an earthquake. Expect traffic and light outages and plan accordingly.
- Open closet and cabinet doors carefully since contents may have shifted.
- Take pictures of any damage to your home, both of the buildings and its contents, for insurance purposes.
- Repair defective electrical wiring and leaky gas connections.
- You should be prepared to take care of yourself and loved ones for a period of seventy-two hours (and possibly longer,

depending on the severity of the earthquake). Seventy-two hours under normal circumstances is how long it typically takes for help to arrive.

- Remember to check on neighbors who may require special assistance, including infants, the elderly, and people with disabilities.
- If power is off, plan meals to use up foods that will spoil quickly or are frozen (food in the freezer should be good for at least a couple of days).
- Pets may not be allowed into shelters for health and space reasons. Prepare an emergency pen for pets in the home that includes a three-day supply of dry food and a large container of water.

Earthquake Mythology

MYTH: Dogs and other animals sense an earthquake and act differently because of it.
TRUTH: We tend to notice things discriminately. You might observe changes in animal behavior prior to an earthquake, but that behavior is not consistent, and sometimes there's no perceptible behavior change prior to an earthquake. Confirmation bias in action. People who perpetuate this myth tend to remember the animal behavior that fits the pattern and forget about the ones that don't.

MYTH: Earthquakes occur during earthquake weather especially when it's hot or dry.
TRUTH: Seriously? Earthquakes occur many miles underground, and can happen at any time, and in any weather.

(Continued)

MYTH: Big earthquakes always occur early in the morning.
TRUTH: Neither weather nor time of day make any difference to when an earthquake will occur.

MYTH: In an earthquake, the ground opens up in a great and immediate rift and swallows cars, houses, and people.
TRUTH: Only in the movies. If the ground opened up like that, there would be no friction and it takes friction for the earthquake to happen. Can earthquakes cause settling and other ground deformation that can include open fissures? Yes, but rarely.

MYTH: The safest place to be in an earthquake is under a doorway.
TRUTH: Not true, for a couple of reasons. First, a swinging door is fairly dangerous. Second, a doorway is no more or less strong than any other place in the house. Third, people go in and out of doors in an emergency, so we expect a doorway will have some urgent traffic.

MYTH: Small earthquakes are deterrents so that the big ones don't happen.
TRUTH: A small quake might temporarily ease stress, but they do not prevent larger tremblors.

MYTH: Earthquakes are becoming more frequent.
TRUTH: Nope. Research shows us that earthquakes of magnitude 7.0 or greater have remained fairly constant throughout the century and have actually decreased in recent years. What may make it seem like there are more

is that today, we have a greater number of seismological centers and instruments capable of locating small earthquakes that went undetected in previous years.

MYTH: There's nothing we can do about earthquakes, so why in the world should we worry about them?

TRUTH: Just because we can't stop earthquakes doesn't mean we shouldn't prepare properly to mitigate the damage they cause. Building modification, education, and preparation are all necessary elements of mitigation. Also, remember that standard homeowners insurance doesn't cover damage from earthquakes.

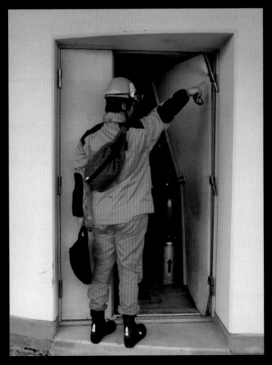

An aid worker after the Haitian earthquake. *Credit: Daisuke Tsuda, creativecommons.org/licenses/by/2.0/.*

The Ten Deadliest Recorded Earthquakes

1. Shensi, China, Jan. 23, 1556. Magnitude 8, approximately 830,000 deaths.
2. Tangshan, China, July 27, 1976. Magnitude 7.5. Official casualty figure is 255,000 deaths. Estimated death toll as high as 655,000.
3. Aleppo, Syria, Aug. 9, 1138. Magnitude not known, about 230,000 deaths.
4. Sumatra, Indonesia, Dec. 26, 2004. Magnitude 9.1, 227,898 deaths.
5. Haiti, Jan 12, 2010. Magnitude 7.0. According to official estimates, 222,570 deaths.
6. Damghan, Iran, Dec. 22, 856. Magnitude not known, approximately 200,000 deaths.
7. Haiyuan, Ningxia, China, Dec. 16, 1920. Magnitude 7.8, about 200,000 deaths.
8. Ardabil, Iran, March. 23, 893. Magnitude not known, about 150,000 deaths.

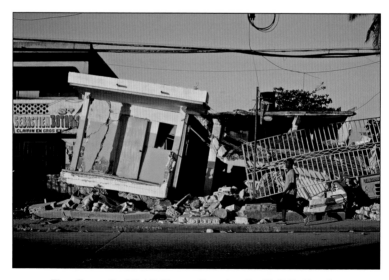

The aftermath of the Haitian earthquake. *Credit: Colin Crowley, creativecommons.org/licenses/by/2.0/.*

- 9: Kanto, Japan, Sept. 1, 192. Magnitude 7.9, 142,800 deaths.
- 10: Ashgabat, Turkmenistan, Oct. 5, 1948. Magnitude 7.3, 110,000 deaths.

CHAPTER NINE

OTHER EXTREME WEATHER

VOLCANO

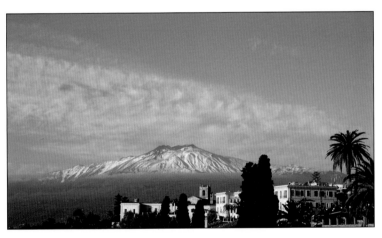

Mount Etna, Sicily. *Credit: Pixabay.*

In the United States, there are fifty active volcanoes. Surprisingly, all over the world, millions of people live near volcanoes. One-hundred-forty thousand people have died as a result of volcanoes over the last five hundred years. The only active volcanoes in America are located in Alaska, Hawaii, and the Pacific Northwest. There are plenty of volcanoes in other states, but they are not active and pose no significant threat.

You might be picturing huge red lava flows destroying entire cities, but these death tolls don't just occur from lava. Gases, toxic smoke, mudflows, pyroclastic projectiles, and even tsunamis are some of the killing results of an eruption. Lava flows are usually due to related causes: collapse of an active lava delta that forms when lava enters a body of water, explosions when lava interacts with water, asphyxiation due to toxic gases, pyroclastic flows from a collapsing dome, and lahars from meltwater.

A volcano is a breach in the earth's surface or crust. Volcanoes erupt when pressure deep inside the earth builds up and is suddenly released. Debris includes lava, dangerous gases, and huge rocks that can be projected into the air and sometimes sail for hundreds of miles. Most volcanoes are dormant and no cause for concern. Volcanoes usually show signs of an impending eruption, which provides time for people located in the immediate vicinity to take precautions.

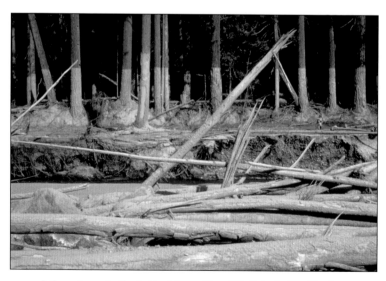

A river channel affected by lahars, Mount St. Helen's, Washington.
Credit: Lyn Topinka, USGS.

Lahars are volcanic mudflows created when water and ash mix. They are fast, deadly, and when they settle, they can be thick and are concrete-like. Pyroclastic flows are avalanches containing hot volcanic gases, ash, and volcanic bombs. On steep volcanoes pyroclastic flows reach speeds of over 100 miles per hour. Lava flows will destroy everything in their path and because of the extreme heat, which will ignite anything and everything. But they move slowly and you'll usually have time to evacuate.

The most dangerous type of volcano is referred to as a supervolcano. A supervolcano usually takes the form of a huge caldera. A caldera is where the land surrounding a volcano collapses following a previous eruption. (Two examples of this can be seen in Valle Vidal in New Mexico and Yellowstone National Park.) Supervolcanoes are different from traditional volcanoes, where an eruption forms a cone-shaped mountain. An eruption of a supervolcano results in catastrophic damage to an entire continent. The chance of such a supervolcano eruption happening today is about one in seven hundred thousand every year.

Preparation

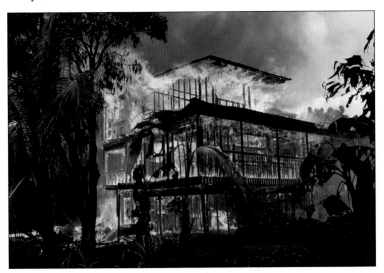

Fire caused by lava flow after the eruption of the Kīlauea Volcano in Hawaii.
Credit: J. D. Griggs, USFS.

Being ready for a volcano is like any other disaster; it requires preparation, education, and operation. Having the proper emergency preparedness kit, having a plan, and knowing what to do before and when a volcano erupts, will greatly improve you and your family's chances of being safe. While some volcanoes erupt without warning, most will provide geological signals that suggest a possible eruption. Warning systems will keep you posted on what might happen.

Know your community's warning system. If you live near a volcano, your community should have a plan in place to warn people that the volcano may erupt. If your community is in any danger, they will likely use a combination of emergency alerts through texts, apps, television, and radio, as well as employing sirens. As soon as you hear a siren, check your phone, turn on the radio, and discover what your local emergency management agency advises. They may advise to stay indoors, keep away from certain areas, or, in extreme cases, evacuate.

Just because you see a plume of debris rising from the volcano, or because you feel an earthquake, doesn't mean the volcano is necessarily going to erupt. Many volcanos burp every so often. That's why you should rely on the local warnings, the experts who know what's going on at the rim. Don't think you can ignore warnings. A volcanic eruption is a scary, unpredictable force. That said, if you are informed about your volcano and you see or feel something, that's your cue to find out more and do so right then.

Most importantly, if you're told to evacuate, do it right away. On the other hand, if you are not instructed to evacuate the area, stay where you are unless you can see immediate danger. Taking to the roads may be more hazardous than staying at home.

Planning

In order to know what to do when a volcano occurs, you need to create a Family Emergency Plan. Sit down with your family members and decide how you will get in contact with each other, where you will go, and what you will do in the event of a disaster or emergency. If a volcano erupts, power could be cut, cell phone service disrupted, and water

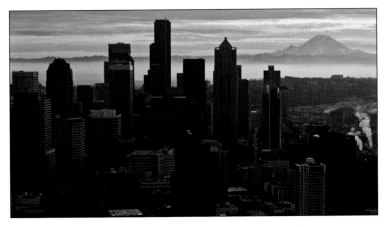

Mt. Rainier, Seattle. *Credit: Lyn Topinka, USGS.*

supply contaminated, so you need to be prepared for these contingencies. Because volcanic eruptions can cause havoc in many different directions, you need to select several alternative routes. These should be the steps of your plan: review evacuation routes; understand emergency alert systems; create evacuation and preparedness plans; prepare emergency kit and food supplies.

<u>Volcano Emergency Supplies List</u>

- Emergency food
- Drinking water
- Flashlights
- Radios
- Sanitation and hygiene supplies
- Emergency blankets
- Phone chargers
- Ziploc baggies to protect against ash
- Extra clothing including long-sleeve shirt, bandana, cap
- A first-aid kit (add different kinds of burn cream, ointment, or gel)
- Blankets and warm clothing
- Cash and change

- Whistle
- Masks (surgical style)
- Particulate filtering face-piece respirators (We recommend the N-95, which is the most common.)
- Manual can opener
- Goggles
- Cash, in case ATMs are down
- A battery-powered radio and fresh batteries
- Hand-cranked radio
- Necessary medications
- A map of the region
- A hazard map of the volcano region. Often, local emergency management agency or U.S. Geological Survey will offer maps that show probable paths of lava flows and lahar (or mud flows) and give estimates for the minimum time it would take a flow to reach a given location. They also divide the area around the volcano into zones, from high-risk to low-risk.

Store at least three days (and preferably two to three weeks') supply of food and water at your home. In the event of an eruption, water supplies may become contaminated. Keep all your supplies in one place. We recommend a storage drum that is sealable, and a backpack or two so you can carry it with you if you need to evacuate.

Sit down with your family and friends and create a household evacuation plan. If the sirens go off, it's easy to panic but if you have a solid plan and everyone is familiar with it, you'll be okay. Come up with one major evacuation route but have two alternative routes. Think about what would happen if you are in your car and the ash clogs the engine. What will you need in your emergency supply list? Who's in charge of the pets in an emergency? It's a good idea to have each person of the household have responsibilities in the plan. Stick a printed checklist on the fridge so you don't forget anything.

If you're visiting a volcano

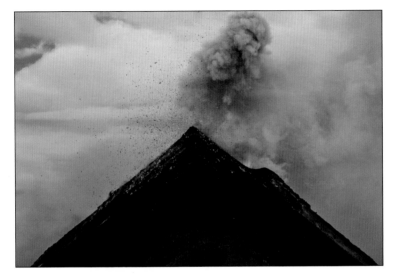

Credit: Pete Johnson.

On one of your future trips, you may find yourself within the eruption zone of an active volcano. Think not? Seattle, Washington. Yellowstone National Park. Oregon, California, Hawaii, Alaska. Italy. Japan. Iceland. Guatemala. Chile. America has 169 active volcanoes (although most are in Alaska) and Europe has sixty. So if you end up near a volcano, it is worthwhile to consider how to survive an eruption because it could happen suddenly.

If you found yourself in a volcanic event, what would you do? Start by letting family and friends know where you'll be. If you are not going with a guide, and you don't come home, they'll know where to begin searching. Did you know many people purposefully visit active volcanoes? Volcanic tours provide a niche tourism for many locales.

Learn about the volcano. Stay informed by listening to the radio or checking the local news. Bring some basic volcano survival gear. Water, first-aid kit, and flashlights are mainstays in any survival kit, but a mask and goggles are must-haves in this kit. If you're hiking near or on the volcano, you'll want to wear a helmet.

When was the last time this volcano erupted? Is it monitored? Would there be any reason for you to expect an eruption? Have there been recent warnings or activity? Additionally, you should still be familiar with the region's warning system. Get familiar with evacuation procedures.

If you're going to be climbing or hiking near the volcano, you should bring a few survival items that will help you survive if you're caught outside without access to shelter. You'll need a respirator and goggles to protect your face and help you breathe. Bring long pants and long-sleeved shirts. Bring a couple of bottles of water in case you become trapped.

Survival

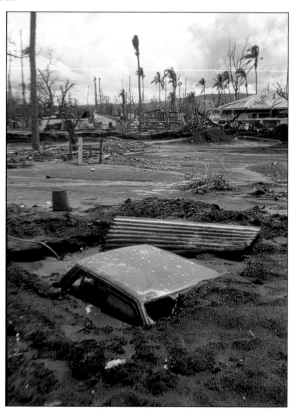

Credit: AusAID,creativecommons.org licenses by 2.0.

The best way to stay safe is to listen to and follow the advice of local emergency management. They will have learned the latest about the volcano from experts and can provide you with the latest information regarding road closures and status reports.

While you are monitoring alerts, be active. Close all windows, doors, and fireplace or woodstove dampers. Turn off all fans and heating and air conditioning systems. Bring pets and livestock into closed shelters. Listen for emergency alerts and do what they say. If you are outdoors. Seek shelter indoors. Stay inside until you hear that it's safe to come out.

If you get caught outdoors, don't stay outdoors. Get inside. You'll have to determine whether you can make it back to your house safely. You might not be able to, and in that case, you'll have planned for this contingency in your emergency plan. Get into a safe building and determine your next course of action. Contact your family members. If you're out in your yard, just go inside. It's understandable to look toward the volcano to see what's going on, but don't gawk for long. Time is of the essence.

If you don't get an evacuation notice, if you decide that you're staying until otherwise determined, go inside to a room with interior walls. Make sure all of your family members and pets are inside. Locate your emergency supplies and bring them with you. If you have time, protect your vehicles by putting them inside the garage.

If you get caught outside and not near shelter, get to higher ground. Watch for flying debris and pyroclastics, which are rocks and debris (often red-hot) sent airborne during an eruption. If there is a projection of smaller pyroclastics, face away from the volcano, hunker down on the ground, and protect your head with your arms, a backpack, or anything else you can find.

One danger that is difficult to avoid, unless you are equipped with a proper gas mask, is exposure to poisonous gases. Volcanoes emit gases, and some of these gases are debilitating and often deadly. If you don't have a proper gas mask, breathe through a respirator, mask, or moist piece of cloth. Volcanic gases are dangerous and are heavier than air. These gases will collect and accumulate near the ground so getting low isn't a good idea. So the idea is that if you sense gases, get away as quickly as possible.

Get to high ground if you can't find shelter. Lava flows, flooding, mudflows (which commonly result from eruptions), and lahars are all deadly and tend to travel through valleys and low-lying areas. Protect your eyes as well. Wear goggles if your mask doesn't cover your eyes. Keep your skin covered with long pants and a long-sleeved shirt. If you see geothermal areas, go around them. Geothermal clues include hot-spots, geysers, or mudpots, and the ground around these is thin. If you fall through, you're going to get burns or worse.

If you decide to drive, grab your emergency kit backpacks. Keep doors and windows closed, the air conditioner off, and don't drive across the path of danger. Follow your evacuation plans, listen to the radio, and watch for unusual hazards in the road. Be prepared to change to your second or third route if needed.

If the predominant result from the eruption is ashfall, this bears close monitoring. Stay inside with windows and doors closed. Because ash is abrasive, wear long-sleeved shirts and long pants. Use goggles to protect your eyes and a mask to protect your breathing. Volcanic ash is composed of particles that are like tiny pieces of glass and will seriously hurt your eyes and lungs. If ash is falling with no end in sight, you may not be able to shelter indoors for more than a few hours, because ash is heavy and the weight of the ash could collapse your roof of your building and/or block air intakes.

Exposure to ash can harm your respiratory (breathing) tract, too. To protect yourself while you are outdoors or while you are cleaning up ash that has gotten indoors, you may steal from your emergency kit or purchase a box of disposable particulate respirators (also known as an air purifying respirator). The N-95 respirator is the most common type of disposable particulate respirator and can be purchased at online or at most hardware stores. Note that disposable particulate respirators do not filter toxic gases and vapors.

Aftermath

The worst might seem like it's over but there are still many hazards facing you from the eruption.

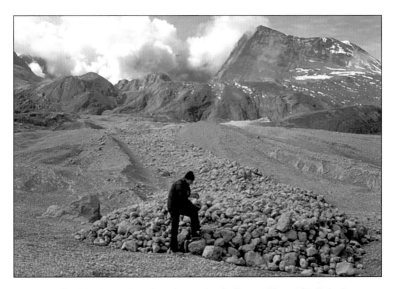

Pumice blocks at the edge of pyroclastic flow at Mount St. Helen's.
Credit: Donald A. Swanson.

First, remain indoors until you're told it's safe to come out. Keep listening to the radio, and if you have service, checking your alerts on your phone and inform family members you are okay.

Stay inside until the ash stops falling. If you do go outside before it's deemed safe, make sure your body is covered from head to toe and that you breathe through a respirator or moistened cloth. Drink only bottled water until the tap water can be determined to be clean. If you see ash in any water or suspect it's invaded the source, avoid drinking it.

Seek medical care for burns or gas right away. Immediate care can be lifesaving. If your eyes, nose, and throat become irritated from volcanic gases and fumes, get away from the area immediately. If your symptoms continue after being away from the volcano for a while, see a doctor.

There is a good chance that if ash falls for many hours, officials might advise evacuating, even after the eruption is over. The danger from roof collapses is real. Stay away from areas with heavy ash fall. Don't walk or drive in areas close to the volcano where a lot of ash has collected. Turn on the radio to find out which areas were most severely affected so you can avoid accidentally ending up in a danger zone.

Areas with high volcanic activity often have designated shelters. If your roof is in danger, you might consider going to a shelter. If your house is getting ash inside it, get to a shelter. You don't want to expose yourself and others to ash and the chemicals in ash. Also, sulfuric acid and other acids may seep into water, so keep checking your water supply.

You want to keep ashfall out of your house or building so close all windows, doors, and any other openings. Turn off all fans and heating and air conditioning systems so you don't bring in or dust up the ash. Your pets need to remain indoors except when they have to go outside for a bathroom break.

Keeping away from ash is especially important for people with respiratory conditions like asthma or bronchitis. Don't drive through areas with heavy ash fall, either. The ash will clog up your engine and ruin it.

Clear ash from your home and property. When you're sure it's safe to go out, you'll need to clear the ash from your rooftop first. Ash is very heavy and can cause roofs to collapse, especially when it's wet. If wind stirs it up, it will be harmful to those who breathe it in. Your vehicles may be covered in ash and it's awfully abrasive so you'll likely end up with paint scratches even if you are careful.

Wear long pants and a long-sleeved shirt, and cover your mouth with a mask so you don't breathe in the ash. You might also want to wear goggles. Shovel the ash into trash bags, then seal them and dispose of them according to your community's recommendations. Don't turn on your air conditioner or evaporative cooler nor should you open up your vents until most of the ash has been cleared away.

Keep your car or truck engine turned off and by all means, avoid driving in heavy ashfall. Driving will stir up ash that can clog engines and stall vehicles. You can easily ruin your engine. If you do have to drive, keep the car windows up and do not operate the air conditioning system. Operating the air conditioning system will bring in outside air and ash.

Replace disposable furnace filters or clean permanent furnace filters. If you discover your drinking water has ash in it, use another source of drinking water, such as purchased bottled water, until your water can be tested or the local authorities give the all clear.

Pay attention to advisories and warnings, and obey instructions from local authorities. For example, if told to stay indoors until local health officials tell you it is safe to go outside, stay indoors. Listen to local news updates for information about air quality, drinking water, and roads. Do not travel unless you have to. Driving in ash is hazardous to your health and your car. Driving will stir up more ash that can clog engines and stall vehicles.

LIGHTNING

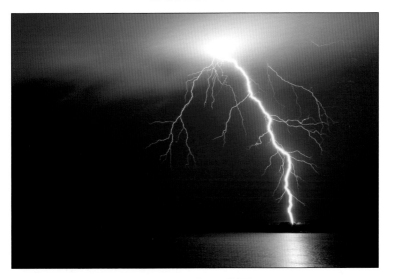

Credit: Kevin Skow, NOAA.

This surprised us, but of all storm-related deaths, lightning comes in at number two, killing more people, on average, in the US than either hurricanes or tornadoes. Only floods kill more than lightning strikes each year. According to the National Weather Service, your typical lightning flash contains a whopping three hundred million volts of electricity. Amazingly, only about 10 percent of those struck by lightning are killed. Ninety percent of the victims survive but many carry lifelong injuries, physical (mostly neurological) and emotional.

In America, lightning strikes kill about one hundred people each year and injure about a thousand. Worldwide, lightning strikes kill twenty-four thousand people and about 240,000 survive lightning. The chances of being the victim from a lighting strike are about one in 600,000.

The best way to survive a lightning strike is to avoid being outdoors in the first place. If you are outside, use the 30–30 Rule. Once you see lightning, start counting. If you can't count to thirty before hearing thunder, get inside proper shelter. Don't go outside until thirty minutes have passed after the last clap of thunder.

So, if you plan to be outside, watch the weather forecast before your go out. Know your local weather patterns, especially in summer months. Plan around the weather to avoid any lightning hazard. Be observant while you are out, and look for clues that thunderstorms are developing. Do you see thickening, darkening clouds? Are the clouds vertical, and are the wind and rain increasing? Lightning can strike with no rain. The rain might be off in the distance but lightning can still occur.

So if you try the 30–30 rule and you determine lightning is likely, seek proper shelter. Don't hesitate, seek shelter immediately. Every second counts.

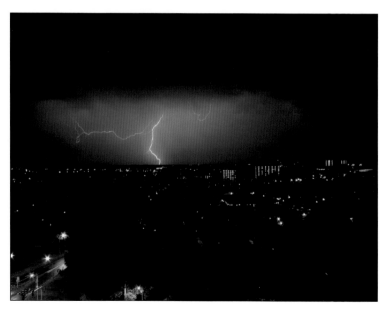

Building

What is proper shelter? The best shelter against lightning is a fully-enclosed, substantially-constructed building, so in other words, the typical house, school, library, or public building. Substantially-constructed means it has wiring and plumbing in the walls so as to divert the electricity from the strike.

Once inside, stay away from any conducting paths to the outside. Stay away from electrical appliances, lighting, and electric sockets, plumbing.

Vehicle

If you can't get to a substantially-constructed building, you might find refuge in a vehicle but not a convertible or car with fiberglass or plastic shells. Avoid contact with conducting paths going outside: close the windows, don't touch the steering wheel, ignition, gear shifter, or radio. Rubber tires and rubber-soled shoes provide virtually no protection from lightning.

Places to avoid

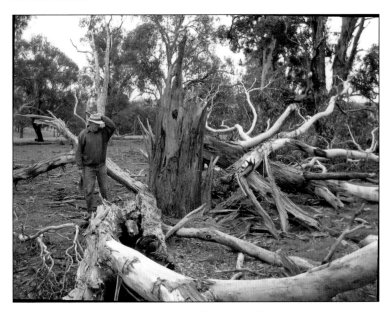

Tree destroyed by lightning strike.

If you can't get to a proper lightning shelter, house, or vehicle, at least avoid the most dangerous locations and activities.

- Avoid higher elevations.
- Avoid wide-open areas (fields and beaches).
- Avoid tall isolated objects like trees, flagpoles, and light posts.
- Avoid being around water sports: boating, swimming or fishing.
- Avoid golfing.
- Avoid unprotected open buildings like picnic pavilions, rain shelters, and bus stops.
- Avoid metal fences and metal bleachers.
- Do not go under trees, either individual or several.

If you're caught outdoors and can't take cover during a lightning storm, do not go to the one tree in an open field. That's the most likely spot for the lightning to strike. Instead seek shelter in a low area like a valley or a ravine. If lightning is imminent, it will sometimes provide you with a few seconds of warning. Sometimes your hair will stand up on end, or your skin will tingle, or light metal objects will vibrate, or you'll hear a crackling sound, or you'll see a blue haze. As a last, desperate measure, get into the lightning crouch. Put your feet together, squat down, tuck your head, and cover your ears.

Lightning First Aid:
If a person is struck by lightning, render assistance immediately. It's a common myth that victims carry an electrical charge but it is not true, and they cannot shock or hurt anyone.

- Call 911.
- Deaths from lightning are from cardiac arrest and stopped breathing at the time of the strike. CPR and mouth-to-mouth-resuscitation are the best ways to recover the victim.
- If you are still in an active thunderstorm and at continuing risk to yourself or your party, move the victim to a safer location.

DUST STORM

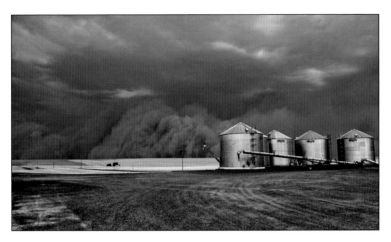

Farm outside of Ritzville, Washington in the midst of a dust storm.
Credit: Susan DeWald, USDA.

If you don't live in the western or southwestern regions of the United States, you may only think dust storms, haboobs, and sandstorms only occur in an Egyptian mummy movie or the deserts of the Middle East. But during the monsoon season of mid to late summer, those in the arid sections of southwest US run the risk of these infrequent but powerful storms.

What is a haboob? A haboob is an intense dust storm that is carried on a weather front. When the storm collapses, when it begins to release precipitation, wind directions reverse, gusting outward from the storm and gusting strongly in the direction of the storm's travel. When this downburst of cold air hits the ground, it blows dust or sand up from the ground, and creates a wall of sediment that precedes the thunderstorm.

This wall of dust can be as wide as fifty to sixty miles (although there have been storms that reach as much as one hundred miles wide) and a mile high. At their strongest, haboob winds often travel at 20 to 60 miles per hour, and the biggest dilemma is that they may approach with little or no warning. You look up and there they are, big, imposing brown walls. Even though the haboob might contain rain, the hot dry air evaporates the water before it reaches the ground. Evaporation cools the air and as a result, accelerates it. Sometimes instead of fronting a rainstorm, haboobs occur when a storm collapses and forms a microburst.

These storms of dust and sand are violent and unpredictable. These high winds lift dirt or sand and unleash a turbulent, suffocating cloud that can reduce visibility to nothing in a matter of seconds and cause property damage, injuries, power outages, travel delays or closures, and even deaths. These storms are especially hazardous to those with eye and respiratory problems. No matter where you live, it's a good idea to know what to do if you see a big dust/sand wall racing toward you.

If you are in a storm-prone area in the western or southwestern United States, you should always be aware that one of these dust storms could occur. Pay attention to dust storm warnings. Dust storms are most likely to occur on hot summer days under certain atmospheric conditions, and meteorologists have gotten good at predicting these storms. Tune in to local TV or radio broadcasts before traveling in hot, dry conditions. If there's a good chance you'll get caught in a dust storm, it's worth thinking about not traveling at all.

Carry a backpack or keep a box in the trunk of your car filled with items you need in the event of a dust/sand storm. Fill the emergency kit with these items:

- A mask designed to filter out small particulates.
- Airtight goggles (eyeglasses won't keep particles out).
- A water supply (bottles of water or a jug).
- A warm blanket because if it's a winter dust storm, things can quickly lead to hypothermia.

You might get caught out away from your house or car and if so, you probably won't have your emergency kit with you. Do not try to outrun one of these dust storms on foot. Wind storms are unpredictable and faster than you, so you could be overtaken if it suddenly changes direction or picks up speed. If you can go into a building or shelter of some kind, do so. If not, get ready to hunker down.

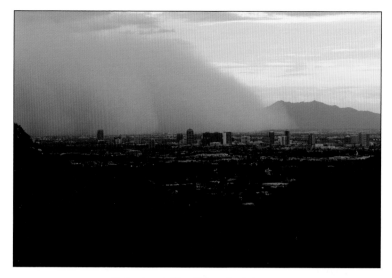

Haboob outside of Phoenix, Arizona.

Cover as much of your body as possible to protect yourself from flying sand. Wind-propelled sand can hurt, but a dust storm's high winds can also carry heavier projectiles too. If you find yourself without shelter, try to stay low to the ground and protect your head with your arms, a backpack, or a purse. Wait out the storm. Don't try to move through the storm because it's too disorienting and too dangerous.

If you have a mask, put it over your nose and mouth. Short of that, use a scarf, bandana, or shirt. A respirator is designed to filter out small particulates, and we recommend this in particular if you have asthma or breathing problems. So if the storm is coming, put it on immediately. Apply a small amount of Vaseline to the inside of your nostrils to prevent drying of your mucous membranes.

Protect your eyes. Airtight goggles offer protection from blowing dust or sand, but eyeglasses don't offer much at all. If you didn't add goggles to your kit, shield your face with your arm or wrap a piece of cloth tightly around your entire head to protect your eyes and ears until the storm passes.

Let's take a different and more-likely scenario:

You're in your car and you see a dust storm from some distance; you may be able to outrun it or detour around it. While some of these storms travel at 60 miles per hour or more, most travel slower than that. You have to make an intelligent decision in trying to outrun a storm, so it is not advisable if you have to put yourself (and your passengers) at risk by traveling at high speeds. If you attempt to outrun it and the storm is catching up with you, stop and prepare for it. Once consumed by the storm, your visibility can potentially be reduced to zero in a matter of seconds. Drive to a safe place where you can take shelter until the storm passes.

Pull the car over and stop. If you're driving and visibility drops to less than two hundred to three hundred feet, it's time to pull off the road. If you are able to pull off somewhere safely, turn off your headlights, roll up the windows and turn off vents that bring outside air in. Turn on your hazard lights, and as you park safely, proceed with caution, and honk your horn periodically.

You want to turn your headlights off so that other drivers don't use your taillights as a guide. You don't want to risk a rear-end collision. If you are pulled off the road and are sitting there with your lights on, someone might think they can follow you. Take cover and stay put. Do not attempt to move about in a blinding dust storm, since you won't be able to see any potential hazards. Heavy rain may follow the dust storm and the combination of rain and dust makes for a messy windshield wiper situation.

ACKNOWLEDGMENTS AND CONCLUSION

We'd like to acknowledge information and resources from FEMA, National Weather Service, National Organization of Atmospheric Administration, American Red Cross, National Hurricane Center, OSHA, National Severe Storms Laboratory, WMO World Weather Information Service, European Severe Storm Laboratory, International Tsunami Information Center, American Meteorological Society, National Center for Atmospheric Research, National Voluntary Organizations Active in Disaster, and the United States Geological Survey.

We wrote this book because we realized how little we knew about the weather disasters we encountered previously. We tirelessly researched how the experts and weather organizations suggested how to prepare, how to survive, and how to navigate the aftermath of numerous disasters. We learned how easy it was to get prepared, to make our emergency plans, to find alternative routes, to build disaster kits, and in fact, preparation became a fun game for us. You can do it too. All it takes is initial impetus and soon, it'll become inclination. That leads to proper preparation and education and those two things greatly increase survival for you and your family. We feel so much more at ease about our chances at surviving the next time we meet up with a tornado or earthquake, haboob, or hurricane.

Weather disasters happen frequently, so the more you are educated about their nature and destructive power, the more you know about how to prepare better for their emergence, and how to survive in the midst of a severe weather event; ergo, the greater odds of survival. We encourage our readers to be active in prevention and education. Don't be a bystander or a victim. You can't fool or stop Mother Nature, but you can prepare for her.